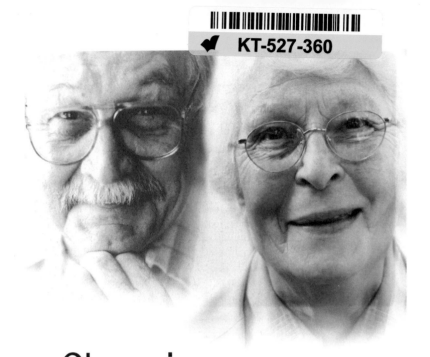

Choosing a
CARE
HOME

MARY V. GOUDGE

howto**books**

Published by How To Books Ltd
3 Newtec Place, Magdalen Road
Oxford, OX4 1RE, United Kingdom
Tel: (01865) 793806. Fax: (01865) 248780
email: info@howtobooks.co.uk
www.howtobooks.co.uk

British Library Cataloguing in Publication Data
A catalogue record for this book is available from the British
Library

Cover design by Baseline Arts Ltd, Oxford
Produced for How To Books by Deer Park Productions,
Tavistock
Typeset by TW Typesetting, Plymouth, Devon
Printed and bound by Cromwell Press, Trowbridge, Wiltshire

NOTE: The material contained in this book is set out in good
faith for general guidance and no liability can be accepted for
loss or expense incurred as a result of relying in particular
circumstances on statements made in this book. Laws and
regulations may be complex and liable to change, and readers
should check the current position with the relevant
authorities before making personal arrangements.

Choosing a
CARE
HOME

If you want to know how . . .

1000 Pocket Positives
Inspiring quotations to enlighten refresh and uplift

Tracking Down Your Ancestors
Discover the story behind your ancestors and bring your family history to life

The Level Guide to the South West
The only personally-assessed tourist guide for those with limited mobility

Writing Your Life Story
How to record and present your memories for friends and family to enjoy

The Self-Help Guide to Making a Will

howtobooks

For full details, please send for a free copy of the latest catalogue to:
How To Books
3 Newtec Place, Magdalen Road
Oxford OX4 1RE, United Kingdom
info@howtobooks.co.uk
www.howtobooks.co.uk

Contents

List of Illustrations

Acknowledgements

Barbara Smith RGN, Deputy Matron, Firtree House, Tunbridge Wells.

Angela Walton, Branch Co-ordinator, Alzheimer's, Eastbourne.

Citizen's Advice Bureau, Eastbourne.

The late Miss Nellie (Sophia) White.

Mrs Jean Lawrence, Miss White's niece.

Mrs Brown, Albert's wife (see Chapter 3).

Mrs Miriam Goss RGN.

Taleb Durgahee RMN, the proprietor of Keller House, Eastbourne.

Michael Baldray, the proprietor of Ennis House, Eastbourne.

Mrs Ruby Smith, Resident, The Hawthornes, Eastbourne.

Special thanks to my husband, Michael, for his support and helpful suggestions regarding this book and for helping out when the printing equipment failed.

Preface

How do you know which care home is the most suitable for your beloved relative or friend? How can you decide where they will be happy and well cared for? This book has been written to help relatives and carers who want to find the right home for their loved one.

Many hospitals complain there is a bed shortage. It is claimed elderly patients cause this because they have nowhere to go after leaving hospital as there is nobody to look after them at home and so they have to stay in hospital. They now need care and help with the activities of daily living such as washing and dressing etc. Some elderly patients are fit enough to be cared for in a residential care home, others need some or total nursing care. There are also elderly patients in the early or middle stages of Alzheimer's disease and others who suffer from a mental illness.

Hospital staff are anxious to free the beds as soon as possible to make way for new patients who need surgery or urgent medical treatment. This puts pressure on care managers and the patient's relatives to find somewhere where their loved one can be cared for on a temporary or permanent basis.

Having been a matron of various nursing homes for many years I have tried to address some of the problems relatives have brought to me for advice when they have come to view the home. They are mostly desperate people trying to find the perfect place where Mum and Dad or another much loved person will soon feel at home, be comfortable, happy and make new friends in addition to maintaining contact with relatives and old friends who visit so faithfully.

You will find this book full of useful information, which, I trust, will make your task easier for you and your loved one. When all the hard work is done and your relative has settled down you will be able to relax and congratulate yourself on a job well done.

Mary Goudge

(1)

Essential Requirements for Residents

To help a new resident feel at home and as happy as they can be in the circumstances, they need to have the basic requirements for an elderly person. These are:

- privacy

- comfort

- warmth

- appropriate food

- kind, understanding staff

- company with people with whom they can make friends

- clean clothing

- toilet training, incontinence pads and pants if required

- help with washing/bathing and toilet

- occupational ploys – hobbies, crafts, etc

- somebody within the staff with whom they can relate

- hand rails along walls, in bathrooms, toilets, etc

- competent care when they are healthy

- competent care during sickness, i.e. headaches, migraines, colds, etc

- a good sized, nicely decorated bedroom with an adequate amount of serviceable furniture including a comfortable bed and chair, wardrobe, chest of drawers, a chair for visitors, commode (if required) curtains and bed linen, towels, etc, hand basin or en-suite facilities.

RESIDENTS WHO NEED NURSING CARE

Due to their physical condition residents who need nursing care need all the above but in addition they also need Registered Nurses on duty at all times who understand:

- their bodily needs

- their illnesses

- their fears and frustrations

- their treatment and nursing care

- how to supervise their nursing care, diet, exercise and drug regime and follow their doctor's instructions regarding their management, to keep them as healthy, happy and active as possible.

RESIDENTS WHO ARE BLIND

There are specific needs for those who are blind.

- They appreciate hand rails, particularly in long corridors.

- They need staff who will take the trouble to guide them to the bathroom or their own room when necessary.

- They need to be seated in a place where there is a clear pathway from their chair to the door without obstructions on the floor that might cause them to trip when walking.

- They require literature and documents printed in Braille, together with 'Talking Books' from the Blind Society.

- Some residents may like to be taken to the local club for the blind if there is one.

A prospective resident who is blind may have a specially trained guide dog whom they would like to keep with them. This would be a matter to discuss with matron and/or the management.

RESIDENTS WHO SUFFER FROM DEAFNESS

Deaf residents may appreciate a loop system if one is fitted in the home.

Deaf residents who could 'sign' would find it helpful if some of the staff were able to sign or willing to learn how to sign. In addition, other residents would need to be taught sign language so that the deaf resident is able to communicate with them.

DISABLED RESIDENTS

Disabled elderly men and women, who are potential residents, need to be assured of the following:

- That there are sufficient numbers of nursing or care staff on duty at all times and that they are capable of caring for them adequately. Also that they will treat them as normal people.

- The home should be well equipped with hoists and any other equipment they need to help them with the functions of daily living.

- There are kind, understanding staff who will encourage the disabled resident to reach their full potential.

- There should be suitable activities, such as table tennis, board games, wheel-chair games, etc.

- They also need plenty of space!

ELDERLY MENTALLY INFIRM RESIDENTS (EMI)

Elderly residents who are burdened with senile dementia, Alzheimer's disease and other mental illnesses are usually nursed in EMI homes (see Chapter 3).

If the resident has lived in a home for a long period of time and goes on to develop dementia they are often allowed to remain in that home during the early stages of the disease, provided they do not become unmanageable, or until a more suitable placement can be made.

TERMINAL ILLNESS

There are many elderly people who have developed a terminal illness such as carcinoma (cancer).

Again their basic needs are the same as any elderly person but in addition they need:

- Hospice nurses who specialise in the care of the terminally ill.

- A specific drug regime to keep any pain at bay.

- Someone they can talk to, to voice their fears, worries and discuss their future.

- Somebody who can help the family come to terms with their loved one's terminal illness, and their subsequent bereavement.

- Somebody who can give them spiritual help.

The patient's doctor or consultant can refer them to a hospice for care. Initially the person is assessed by the hospice staff. Drugs (medications) for pain and discomfort are prescribed and given until the person is virtually pain free. The patients are then usually allowed to return home but are visited by a hospice nurse on a regular basis.

If deterioration takes place, arrangements are made for the patient to be re-admitted to the Hospice for further assessment and treatment. The patient, provided they are well enough, is allowed home after each stay in the hospice as long as they are able.

The hospice nurse will advise the family, the doctor and hospice staff as to the progress or deterioration of the patient. They may suggest different methods of care or ways of helping the patient.

The hospice nurse not only looks after the patient but also cares for the family, throughout their loved one's illness and the family's bereavement. The hospice movement provides care, help, hope and freedom from pain.

Some nursing homes, in conjunction with the local hospice, reserve beds for residents with a terminal illness. The hospice nurses discuss the ongoing treatment, drug regime and care with the resident's doctor and the matron before it is put into practice.

Chronic illnesses such as multiple sclerosis or muscular dystrophy are usually nursed in a suitable nursing home but are sometimes cared for in a hospice.

RESPITE CARE

If you are nursing a relative or friend with a chronic illness, you can apply to the social services to give you a break by asking them to find a home which caters for patients needing respite care whilst the carer has a rest. It may be possible for your relative or friend to be admitted for one or two weeks depending on the needs of yourself, the carer, your relative and vacancies.

This type of home does not generally provide nursing care and whoever is admitted should be almost self-caring even though they may need supervision. The temporary residents are well looked after, usually enjoy their stay and look upon it as a holiday.

However, if your relative needs nursing or psychiatric care, they would be admitted to an appropriate home for respite care. You would need to discuss this arrangement with their care manager. Depending on your relative's financial status, they may be asked for a contribution towards their care.

Assessing Your Relative's Needs

MAKING NOTES

It is helpful if you make notes of all the various pieces of information you learn about your relative. Thus new knowledge will help you find the right care home for them.

The matron of the home you have chosen will need to know as much about the prospective resident as possible. Any information you are able to give will help them make their own assessment.

It will also help the matron to instruct the nurses in their general care of your relative if they decide to admit them.

Use an exercise book to keep all your notes together. The first page might be kept for their personal details.

PERSONAL DETAILS

Even though you probably know most of your relative's personal details it is a good idea to write them down so that they don't fly from your memory when you're asked for them.

Some of the questions you may be asked:

- Your relative's full name and date of birth.

- Their current address and telephone number.

- Their status, for example whether they are retired.

- Whether you are the next of kin and if not who is.

- The next of kin's address and telephone number.

- Past and current illnesses.

- Current medications.

- Whether they are mobile, use a walking aid or are confined to a wheelchair.

- If they suffer from any pain, its severity and cause, if known.

- The matron will want to know the name of their doctor, the address and phone number of the surgery.

- The date, time and place of any hospital appointments which may have been arranged for your relative.

- The matron may be interested in your relative's past employment or profession because this can sometimes be contributory to the cause of some of their current problems.

If you are not next of kin you may still be asked for your own address and telephone number so that you can be contacted if necessary, regarding admission arrangements.

PHYSICAL NEEDS

Try to establish how your relative copes with daily living, and whether they have any help from social services such as a home help.

Try to find out in which way they are incapacitated. Are they mobile at all, or do they have any appliances such as a walking aid to help them? Some people have trolleys so they can transport their food and drink or other things and use it to help support themselves at the same time.

If they have been lame for some years they may have calipers for their legs which have to be strapped on each day. They may have a manual or battery operated wheelchair.

Food and drink

Is your relative able to prepare their own meals, take their food and drink to the table, sit down, eat and drink without help?

Some people need special cutlery and drinking cups to help them eat and drink. Although these are supplied where necessary, they may prefer to take their own with them rather than have to get used to the ones provided.

Do they suffer from any illness that requires a special diet, such as diabetes? Food allergies also have to be considered so alternative foods or special diets can be prepared for them. The matron needs to know in order to instruct the chef and ask them to visit the new resident.

Using the toilet
Can your relative get to and from the toilet by themselves? Sometimes it takes too long for this to be accomplished and elimination takes place before the toilet is reached. If the matron knows about this problem arrangements can be made for a resident to be taken to the toilet at regular intervals before they are desperate to eliminate. Hopefully this will solve the problem.

Some people are incontinent of urine which is not always improved with treatment and tends to worsen with age. Others are doubly incontinent and need to wear incontinence pads all the time. In most homes these are supplied free of charge but in others a charge may be made.

Incontinence is an embarrassing affair for any adult and they sometimes try to hide it. However, the matron does need to know and will be quite used to this situation and will discuss the matter with you.

Pain, current illness and prognosis
Take notes about the amount of pain, if any, your relative suffers from. It would be useful to find out what medication they take to keep them relatively pain free. Severe pain is sometimes treated at a pain clinic, to which their doctor would refer them if it was thought necessary.

If they have a current illness you might like to see their doctor and ask how best to help them. The doctor may be willing to discuss your relative's future management with you.

Pressure sores

A few people who are not really able to care for themselves any longer develop pressure sores on their sacrum, elbows, heels and other places, in fact anywhere where there is constant unrelieved pressure on the body. Sacral sores can be made worse by incontinence. The matron will want to know if your relative is suffering from any skin condition including pressure sores so the problem can be assessed by the doctor and treated.

Breathing

Many people suffer from breathing difficulties, such as emphysema or severe asthma. If your relative has this kind of difficulty, they may have been prescribed oxygen (as directed) and will have an oxygen cylinder near to hand. They may need to take this with them but usually the home can get a replacement on prescription. You would need to check this out with the matron.

Speech, hearing and sight

Being unable to speak coherently with clear diction is not an illness but may be due to congenital or life-long deafness. Today deaf children are fitted with hearing aids and taught to speak but 80 years ago many deaf children had little or no help at all. They grew up completely deaf and with few communication skills. Speech difficulties can also be caused by a Stroke (CVA), shock, trauma or a lack of speech training in childhood.

Impaired sight can mostly be improved with spectacles or surgery, removal of cataracts is very successful. Unfortunately, not everybody benefits from treatment and their sight deteriorates in time.

Make a note of hearing aids and batteries your relative has if they are deaf, the number of pairs of glasses they may have and any other aids your relative uses.

PSYCHOLOGICAL NEEDS

Does your relative suffer from any mental illness such as senile dementia or Alzheimer's disease? If they do they will probably be happier if they are placed in an EMI (elderly mentally infirm) home where the nurses are trained to care for residents with this type of illness. However, you, as their relative, may find it distressing at first (see Chapter 3).

Personality

The dictionary tells us that personality is the distinctive character or qualities of a person as distinct from other people.

Everybody has been created in a unique fashion. Everybody has a different personality. This needs to be taken into consideration when looking for a home where they will be cared for.

Some people are extroverted whilst others are introverted. Some people always seem to be anxious whilst others are placid. At this stage it is wise to make notes of all these things. When you start to search for the best home it is very easy to forget details such as these.

Fear

Many elderly people have developed fears over the years, often ones that have developed from incidents in their earlier life.

Many elderly people develop a fear of going into a residential home of any kind. Their main fear seems to be their loss of independence and privacy. If these fears can be determined and allayed, it will help the person to replace fear with positive thinking and anticipation.

Attitude

Attitude is a settled opinion or way of thinking. Body language and behaviour can often reflect a person's attitude.

You may already have noticed that your relative has a settled opinion towards the way in which procedures should be carried out, for instance, the way their home is kept clean, or the way food should be prepared and cooked.

They may have an ingrained attitude towards some people, maybe because they are of a different race, or different religion. However wrong we may feel these attitudes are they can be difficult to change. A lot of tolerance and patience is needed, especially if their attitude towards residential care is negative (see Nellie's Story at the end of the chapter).

Likes and dislikes

Everybody has likes and dislikes and your relative is no exception. If you know of anything they dislike tell the staff at their new residence. It would help to avoid any upsets.

SPIRITUAL NEEDS

Many people attend a place of worship and take Communion on a regular basis. It is a part of their life.

The matron may have arranged for interdenominational church services conducted by a local vicar or pastor in one of the communal rooms on a regular basis, perhaps once a month. Some homes have services for other faiths, if required, conducted by the appropriate spiritual leader, eg priest, rabbi, etc.

If your relative is well enough and makes their desires known, they will, if possible, be taken into the service. They can request a visit from their own spiritual leader who may be able to arrange for them to be taken to their normal place of worship by the members, providing:

◆ your relative is well enough;

◆ their doctor and person in charge at the time agree;

◆ arrangements are made beforehand.

HOBBIES AND ACTIVITIES

Some elderly people still have hobbies. Some like craft work, others might like gardening, reading, philately, music, etc.

Homes which cater for elderly residents usually have a programme of activities including supervised gentle exercise to help maintain mobility. Check with your relative's doctor whether it is advisable for them to participate in this activity, particularly if they have had a pacemaker fitted. If your relative has a hobby or a favourite occupation make a note of it.

One lady chose to live in a residential home for the elderly, and liked to play Scrabble. There was none available in the home at the time but the manager bought one for her use.

However, not all managers have the authority to go and buy things like Scrabble so the onus is often laid on the next of kin to provide board games or craft materials for the resident.

FROM HOME TO HOME!

While your relative lives in their own home, they have their own routine. This will obviously change when they are admitted to a residential care or nursing home.

♦ They will not have to do any housework, laundry or cooking.

♦ They will have help with bathing, washing and dressing if required.

They may find time passes slowly until they get used to the new routine.

Try to get them interested in the programme of activities provided in their new home. It will help to pass the time and they will make new friends. They will learn new hobbies and settle down more quickly.

LEAVING THEIR SPOUSE

Not all elderly people are single or widowed, many are still living in a happy and loving relationship with the person they married when they were younger. It is very hard for both parties to be separated after years of being together. The wife may feel guilty she has 'left' her husband even though it's not her fault. The husband may not even know how to boil an egg or do the shopping because his wife has always cooked and shopped for both of them. It is especially hard if there are no children or other relatives to help out. Whether it is the husband or wife that is admitted to a home they will need a lot of reassurance and tender loving care.

LEAVING A PARTNER

For those who have lived together with a friend for companionship or in a homosexual relationship separation is equally as traumatic. They may have lived together for many years and have become a partner to each other.

If one is admitted to a care home for life both of the friends will grieve. Both will need help and understanding and possibly counselling.

CARE MANAGER (SOCIAL WORKER)

If your relative currently has any help from social services they will be under the care of a care manager. If they do not have a care manager contact your local social services before choosing a nursing home for your loved one. You will be able to find the telephone number in your local phone book. Social services will make an appointment for you to see a care manager to discuss your relative's needs and future management.

DEALING WITH DEATH

None of us, including our loved ones, live for ever. When bereavement happens it's difficult to think of things such as funeral arrangements and impossible if you are on holiday when it occurs.

Many care establishments ask for the wishes of their residents and next of kin as soon as arrangements are made for the resident's admission.

You may need to gently probe to establish your relative's wishes. Listed below are ten things you and the matron will need to know.

1. Has any part of your relative's body been donated and to whom?

2. Has their body been donated for medical science? If so who is to be contacted when the event occurs?

3. Their religion.

4. Which place of worship would they like the service to be held in, if any?

5. It is essential that you know your relative's religion. Followers of the Catholic faith must receive last rites from a priest prior to death; Muslim, Hindu and

Jewish faiths, amongst others, have certain rituals that have to be followed before or immediately after a person dies.

6. Whether they would prefer to be interred or cremated. If cremation, where would they like to have the ashes scattered?

7. Have they a personal preference regarding which funeral director they would like used?

8. They may have contributed to a funeral plan, in which the funeral is wholly or partly paid for. You will need to obtain the papers, either to keep yourself or to photocopy for reference purposes.

9. Some people like to arrange their own funeral service in advance but others would prefer to leave it to those left behind.

10. Would they like flowers or prefer to have donations sent to a charity of their choice?

CHECKLIST

- Have you established how your relative copes at home on their own?

- Do you know whether your relative has donated any parts of their body after death?

- Have you made notes of their abilities, general health, allergies, likes and dislikes, etc?

NELLIE'S STORY
Interviews with Miss Nellie White

Nellie White was 102 years old and had been a committed Christian for almost a century.

Her body was very frail, she couldn't walk but could transfer from wheelchair to her chair with very little or no help. Her sight was so poor she was almost blind and she wore a hearing aid, but her mind was as active as ever and her memory was razor sharp.

Nellie lived alone in a first floor flat helped by relatives, carers and friends. Carers called in at 7.30am to help her with her toilet and dressing, before getting her breakfast. They called in at midday to give her lunch, again about 5pm to see to her needs and give her tea, and lastly at about 8.15pm to give her a tiny dish of bread and milk and then get her ready for bed.

Nellie had two nieces, Florrie, who was 85 and Jean who was retired but younger than Florrie. They both visited their Aunt frequently. Jean often took her to her own home for a few days. She always slept on the settee in the same room to be on hand if her aunt needed anything. This exhausted her. Sometimes she stayed at her Aunt's flat but could only manage a night or two, before she got too tired and needed to go home and rest.

Eighteen months ago Nellie bought an electrically operated recliner chair which she liked using. Some while ago she found it too uncomfortable to sleep in her bed, so she lay awake all night. It became difficult for her to transfer from her bed into her wheelchair to go to the bathroom. Because of her difficulties she chose to sleep in the recliner.

She could transfer from the recliner into her wheelchair and propel herself to just outside the bathroom. With the aid of strategically placed grab rails, she somehow managed to drag herself into the bathroom and onto the toilet. This caused everybody great concern in case she fell and was unable to use her 'life-line' alarm to obtain help.

Despite all her difficulties Nellie was adamant that she would not go into residential care of any kind.

One Sunday evening I felt led to tell my dear friend Nellie how concerned we all were, pointing out that none of us were able to stay every night with her, especially as it was now necessary for her to have continuous help on a permanent basis. There were five of us there at the time and we expected her to be very upset at my suggestion.

Much to everybody's surprise and relief Nellie said, 'I'm praying about it.'

One evening Nellie told me something of her background.

'I had five sisters but I'm the only one left now. I used to live with my sister in a two bed-roomed flat on the next floor, until she died. After that I moved down here into this smaller flat and I've been here more than 20 years now.'

'Nellie, how do you manage at night when there's no one to help you?' I asked.

'It's very difficult but I ask God to help me and He always gives me the strength.'

'What are you going to do when your nieces go on holiday?'

'Social services have arranged for me to have respite care for a week. Will you come and take me there in your car?'

When Nellie returned to her flat after her week in respite care I asked her, 'Did you enjoy your stay in The Laurels?'

'Yes, everybody was so kind. Nothing was too much trouble for them.'

'Nellie, why don't you want to go into a residential care home permanently?'

'I wouldn't be able to do as I want, I wouldn't be able to go to church, I'd lose my independence and I'd have to give up my home. They might not let me play my piano.'

'Don't you think that might be better than falling and hurting yourself when you're alone?'

'Well, I will be going back into The Laurels when Jean goes away again in four weeks' time. I like it there.'

'What about during the meantime, before you go, neither Jean nor Vera (her friend) can manage to sleep here all the time?'

'Oh, Sarah (aged 93) will stay with me and wheel me to the bathroom during the night.'

A few weeks later Nellie's niece was asked to go Italy. Social services arranged for Nellie, at her request, to have respite care again but unfortunately not in the usual home. We had all heard good reports of this home and Nellie was quite happy about the arrangement.

I took her home from church the following Sunday evening. We chatted together as I prepared her supper.

'When I get back from Knight's Court Jean will still be away. I'm going to see if I can stay an extra week' she told me.

'Good idea, you won't be on your own at night then will you?'

'No. I pray every night the Lord will help me and He does but I really can't manage on my own now. I am praying about it though, I'm sure He will give me the answer.'

I saw Nellie a week later. She was different.

'What has happened?' I asked her. She told me the story.

'When I was 15 I used to sing a song at church. I haven't heard or thought about these words since I was a girl. It came into my mind the other day. Do you know it?

'If Jesus goes with me, I'll go anywhere
T'is heaven in me, wherever I be.

When He is near. I count it a privilege here
His cross to bear.
If Jesus goes with me, I'll go anywhere.

'Fancy the Lord putting that into my mind after 87 years! It was an answer to my prayer. I've decided that if Jesus will go with me I'll go into a care home.'

Nellie was placed in Knight's Court, a short-term care home, temporarily.

'It's wonderful here. They couldn't treat me any better if I was the Queen! I'm going to stay here until my care manager finds me a place in a residential care home. I'm hoping to get a place in The Oaks. Everybody says it's lovely there' she told me when I visited.

'I think you've made the right decision Nellie', I replied.

Nellie waited for an assessment and a new permanent placement. She was quite content.

Three weeks later
Eventually, Nellie was assessed by a care manager and a trained nurse. She had set her heart on going into a residential care home but it was decided she needed nursing care. She was very distressed. She really didn't want to go into a nursing home but would have been content to live in a residential care home.

Despite all the care Nellie received her condition began to deteriorate.

Jean and Florrie asked Nellie's care manager to find a place for Nellie. There was a shortage of nursing home beds at the time, however a room was found for her in a local nursing home. Within hours Nellie had been assessed by the matron of The Heritage and she was transferred.

Every care was given to her.

Jean and Florrie spent day and night with her, she was never left alone until she died a few days later.

Lessons to be learned
Nellie was 102 years old. She needed somebody with her every night to wheel her into the bathroom and help her transfer from the wheelchair to the toilet. Afterwards, of course she needed to get back to her chair and be made comfortable again. Unfortunately, the financial resources were not available to provide her with carers who could stay all night.

Nellie was quite happy to have temporary respite care because she knew she could go back to her flat with all her own things around her and the many visitors who came in to help her.

She was reasonably happy when she thought she was well enough to be cared for in a residential care home. In fact she hoped there would be new companions for her to talk to and activities in which she could participate.

Nellie started to give up when she was told she needed nursing care. She knew she could no longer care for herself in her own flat. Even though she knew she could not be left alone at night she didn't really want to go into a nursing home. She could only have her oxygen as prescribed by the doctor instead of having the amount she felt she needed. She felt she would be too regimented, she would not be able to live her life as she wanted to.

$$\left(\begin{array}{c}3\end{array}\right)$$

Dementia, Alzheimer's Disease and Care Homes

As people grow older there is a greater risk of dementia or Alzheimer's disease developing. It not only affects the patient themselves but also the whole family and friends.

DEMENTIA

Dementia is a brain disorder that seriously affects a person's ability to carry out the activities of daily living. Dementia is progressive and incapacitating if it occurs in the earlier years the mental deterioration advances more rapidly and is more severe than if it starts in later years. In people over 65 years old early symptoms resemble the forgetfulness of ageing. Many people worry they are becoming demented.

The earliest symptoms

A close relative may notice failing memory and initiative. The person may become irritable. The loss of memory is a gradual process, patients can often remember incidents in their past but cannot remember recent happenings. This is called short-term memory loss.

After a time the relatives may notice the person does not understand what is said to them and they appear to have lost interest in their former activities and hobbies.

Not all signs of confusion or impaired capacity in the elderly are due to senile dementia. There may be another cause which when treated can reverse the condition. If your relative has this problem persuade them to see their doctor who will probably refer them to a geriatrician (a consultant who specialises in the care of elderly people). They will give advice on the patient's management and/or may refer them to a clinic, sometimes known as a memory clinic. The patient will be seen by a consultant, who not only specialises in the care of the elderly person but also in memory loss, its cause and management.

The most common form of dementia in elderly people is caused by Alzheimer's disease.

ALZHEIMER'S DISEASE

This disease involves the parts of the brain which control thought, memory and language. Research is ongoing and although much has already been done neither the medical profession nor the scientists know the cause of this disease. So far, no cure has been found.

The disease was first recognised in 1906 by Dr Alzheimer, a German doctor, who discovered abnormal changes in the brain during an autopsy (post-mortem) of a lady who had died of an unusual mental illness. Since then scientists have found that in this disease nerve cells die in greater numbers than normal, in areas of the brain which are vital to memory and other mental abilities. They also noticed that there are lower levels of some of the chemicals in the brain necessary for carrying messages between the nerve cells.

Alzheimer's disease usually begins after the age of 60 and the risk rises with age but this disease is not a normal part of ageing.

What causes Alzheimer's disease?
The cause is unknown at present but there are several factors which may be contributory.

Age
◆ The risk factor increases in people over 65.

◆ As people reach their seventies and eighties the risk factor increases. This is known as 'late onset Alzheimer's disease'.

Family history
There is a rare form of Alzheimer's which is familial. It usually occurs between the ages of 30 and 60 years of age and is inherited. This has led scientists to believe genetics may play a role in some cases.

However, the more common form which occurs later in life shows no sign of being inherited.

Deposits
Autopsies carried out on people who died of Alzheimer's disease in the 1970s showed accumulations of isolated aluminium in some areas of the brain in addition to the changes in the nerve cells which was discovered in 1906. These changes cannot be seen whilst the patient is still living.

Aluminium
It was thought at one time that deposits of aluminium in the brain were contributory to Alzheimer's disease but this has now been largely discounted.

Other factors?
Scientists are continuing with their research and are currently researching education, diet and environment to establish if any of these are factors in the onset and development of the disease.

Protective factors
There is, however, some evidence that physical, mental and social activities may work as protective factors against Alzheimer's disease.

Signs and symptoms
◆ Slow onset.

◆ Mild forgetfulness, patients may have difficulty in remembering recent events, the names of people they know – even their family members.

◆ Patients may not be able to solve simple problems or do simple sums which may cause minor difficulties. However, it's not usually serious enough to cause alarm.

◆ Most people will not suspect anything is wrong at this stage.

◆ The person may begin to forget how to do simple tasks such as combing their hair or cleaning their teeth.

◆ They can't seem to think clearly.

- They may ask the same question repeatedly, or repeat an activity, such as washing their hands, because they have forgotten they have asked the question or washed their hands already.

- Problems arise with speaking, reading, writing and understanding.

- As the disease develops the changes are more pronounced and more easily noticed. At this stage either the person or a family member, on their behalf, will seek medical advice.

- As time passes the person may become anxious, agitated, aggressive, suffer with insomnia and depression.

- They may become wanderers – going out and getting lost.

- Eventually they will need total care.

At the present time an accurate diagnosis can only be made after the person dies and a post-mortem is performed. Diagnosis therefore can only be possible or probable.

On examination the doctor will ask:

- for details of the patient's current general health;

- past medical problems including any surgical procedures which have been carried out;

- the time when the onset of the patient's growing difficulty in performing the tasks of daily living first became apparent.

Memory tests will be carried out such as:

◆ problem-solving;
◆ attention span;
◆ counting;
◆ language.

The following medical tests may be given:

◆ blood tests;
◆ urine analysis;
◆ analysis of spinal fluid;
◆ brain scan.

Sometimes these tests reveal other causes of the symptoms such as:

◆ thyroid problems;
◆ drug reactions;
◆ depression;
◆ brain tumours;
◆ diseased blood vessels.

Some of these can be treated successfully.

How long is the course of the disease?

Alzheimer's is a slow disease and the length of time it takes from diagnosis to the end varies. On average, these patients live for approximately eight to ten years after diagnosis but they can live up to 20 years after a possible or probable diagnosis.

Most doctors believe that Alzheimer's disease is incurable but some doctors and nutritionists believe that this disease is a physical reaction to poisonous substances present in the body and in the environment. It has been suggested that some people are sensitive to processed foods, mercury vapour from amalgam dental fillings and plaque build-up in their arteries, which may be a factor in the onset and progression of this disease.

In the book *All your Health Questions Answered* by Maureen Kennedy Salaman published by MKS Inc. (USA) the author tells a story of a man who was diagnosed as having Alzheimer's disease. He was told the disease was incurable and that he had approximately seven years to live. He didn't accept this verdict. He researched the disease and came to his own conclusions regarding his diet, exercise, the poisons in his body and his way of life etc. After four long, painful years he had yet another brain scan. Much to his doctor's astonishment the 'Alzheimer's' had been reversed.

As Alzheimer's disease can only be accurately diagnosed by a post-mortem we don't really know whether this was a miracle or whether the man really did manage to reverse the disease or whether he had Alzheimer's disease in the first place.

The full story of this man is told in his book *Beating Alzheimer's* (Avery Publishing Group, New York 1991).

CARE FOR PATIENTS WITH ALZHEIMER'S DISEASE

In England people diagnosed with Alzheimer's disease are usually cared for by the family in their own home in the early stages. There comes a time however, as the disease progresses and the behavioural pattern becomes more difficult to cope with, when carers find they can no longer cope with their relative's forgetfulness, odd behaviour and possible aggressiveness.

If you are a carer in this situation contact your relative's care manager and seek advice. They will be able to tell you which kind of home would be most suitable for them and give you a list of appropriate homes.

An EMI home (elderly mentally infirm)

An EMI home is usually the home where residents with dementia or Alzheimer's disease are cared for. A person suffering in this way will be happier in this type of home than in a nursing home. There are Registered Mental Nurses (RMNs) who are specially trained to care for residents with this kind of illness on duty at all times. They know how best to help and care for the residents.

I visited such a home where 15 people suffering from dementia and Alzheimer's disease are being cared for. The first thing I saw was the notice on the wall outside stating it is a residential home for the elderly. I asked the proprietor about this and he told me he wanted everything to be as normal as possible for the residents.

While I was waiting for the proprietor, Mr Durgahee, to arrive I sat in the lounge with the residents. They appeared to be happy and well cared for.

According to the weekly activity programme it was a games afternoon but most of the residents wanted to watch a film on the television which lasted an hour. During this time they were given a cup of tea and cake. After the film ended the residents played Scrabble and other board games.

The proprietor and staff frequently take the residents out to places of interest in the minibus. They are even taken to the theatre on occasions.

On days when they are 'at home' they can join in the scheduled activity for that day, play bingo, cards, or something else they enjoy doing. Relatives and friends are allowed to visit at any time to chat with their loved ones and the other residents if they wish.

Doctors monitor their patients' progress or deterioration and prescribe drugs as appropriate but these are kept to a minimum.

Residential care homes for elderly folk with a mental disorder

These homes cater for elderly residents who suffer from such illnesses as depression or schizophrenia.

One of the homes I visited has 40 residents. They have a weekly activities programme and are taken out in the minibus to various places of interest. There were three recreation rooms, one of which was kept for smokers; smoking is not allowed in the bedrooms due to fire precautions. The dining room was set out with ten round tables with pretty table cloths and small vases of flowers. The room was bright and cheerful.

The residents were chatty, one young man told me he was writing a book and it was going to be a best seller!

Some of the residents need to have regular medication administered by injection, usually fortnightly or monthly. The Community Psychiatric Nurse (CPN) visits frequently to monitor the residents, to give advice if necessary and to give the injections as they become due.

MRS BROWN'S STORY

Mrs Brown was distraught and told me what had happened.

I couldn't care for Albert, my husband, any longer. He is a large man and was diagnosed as suffering from Alzheimer's disease three years ago. In the early stages it wasn't too bad. He was forgetful, but now he can't remember where he is most of the time.

It was a gradual process but there came a time when I had to sew name and address labels in all his clothes in case he went out without me and got lost. He would sneak out when I was upstairs, making the beds. The police have brought him home several times.

Sometimes I had to get some shopping. On this particular day I needed milk, bread and eggs. I couldn't get anyone to sit with Albert not even for half an hour. I thought he would be alright if I locked the door and slipped down to the corner shop. He was sleeping in his chair at the time. I was only a few minutes but by the time I got back he had woken up and decided to do some cooking!

You've never seen such a mess in your life. Everything had been pulled out of the cupboard, flour, salt, sugar, tea, syrup all poured out and spilt on the floor. I saw the mess and wept. Albert got so angry he frightened me.

The strain of the last three years was too much for me. I phoned the doctor. When he came he was concerned because he thought I was going to have a breakdown and urged me to phone Albert's care manager.

By the time I managed to get hold of Mrs Kemp (Albert's care manager) the doctor had already spoken to her and asked if Albert could be taken into respite care as soon as possible. Mrs Kemp came to see me within the hour. She had found a place for Albert at The Gables, an EMI home, a short bus ride away.

Mrs Kemp told me we would have to have a financial assessment but the information I had given her suggested I wouldn't have to dip into our meagre savings to contribute towards Albert's care.

I hastily packed a case with his clothing and put all his medications ready to take with us. A minibus from the home arrived. Albert would be away for two weeks' respite care so I could rest.

It was wonderful to feel so free again after Albert had been admitted to The Gables but after all the clearing up and household chores had been done I felt guilty. Guilty because I wasn't able to look after him anymore. I couldn't face having him back again.

A week later I contacted Mrs Kemp again and told her I couldn't cope with Albert any more.

She was very kind and said, 'I will see what can be done.'

The financial assessment had been carried out before I heard that Albert could stay as a permanent resident at The Gables.

I went to see him, he seemed content and as happy as he could be. I felt guilty and saddened that after 40 years of marriage I could no longer cope with my dear husband. I visited him almost every day and broke my heart when Albert did not know my name or recognise me. But it came as a great relief to know he was in good hands and well looked after.

(4)

Different Kinds of
Residential Care Homes

BUILDINGS

Conversions

Different types of buildings can be converted into care
homes. For instance, older properties are sometimes
converted for the use of elderly people needing residential
care, nursing care or because they may need specialised
care.

Some of these converted buildings were once manor
houses, part of a country estate, set in beautiful grounds.
The rooms tend to be spacious with high ceilings.

Bear in mind that the cost might be higher than usual. If
the home is in a country area, public transport could
cause a problem.

Buildings which have been converted or extended often
have a mixture of modern and older-style accommodation.

Purpose-built

Purpose-built properties are homes which have been
specially built to cater for the needs of elderly people.

Registration

All buildings and accommodation aimed at providing any type of care will have been subject to planning permission and rigorous inspections during the conversion of a property or the building of an extension.

Before the registration certificate can be given:

- The premises are inspected again to ensure rooms are the correct size and suitable for their designated purpose of caring for elderly residents whether they need residential care, nursing care, or for any other type of residential care.

- The premises are also inspected by the fire officer regarding fire doors, fire hazards, fire fighting equipment i.e. fire extinguishers, fire hoses, fire blankets, etc.

WARDEN CONTROLLED FLATS

Warden controlled flats are not classed as care homes but they deserve a mention here.

A warden is employed to ensure that residents who live in these flats are well enough and able to care for themselves on a daily basis, and to answer any emergency calls when they are on duty.

Each flat has a call bell or intercom which rings in the warden's office if they are in need of help during office hours. In order that the residents can call for help when the warden is off duty the residents are usually advised to hire a 'press-button-gadget' (sometimes called 'life line').

This is a call bell, usually in the form of a pendant, which residents can wear round their neck. When the bell is pressed it rings in an office in another building often miles away in another town or city. The person who answers will call the resident's next of kin and advise them of the problem.

RESIDENTIAL CARE HOMES

Men and women are admitted to these homes for care such as bathing, meals, washing, etc. However, these homes are not usually allowed to admit anybody who needs nursing care. Most of these homes employ care assistants who work under the direction of the matron or manager. Usually a suitable weekly activities programme is arranged and even trips to the shops or various places of interest, for those residents who are interested.

The ratio of staff to residents may be lower than in a nursing home because the residents are usually able to do more for themselves. They are not expected to make their beds, do any housework or cooking but they should be able to carry out most of their own personal care when they are admitted.

The snag is that if any resident becomes ill and needs nursing care they may have to be transferred to a nursing home. Initially such a move often upsets the resident and they will need a lot of comforting and help until they learn the routine and make new friends in their new abode.

NURSING HOMES

Nursing homes have a higher ratio of staff to residents than residential care homes because the residents are less able than clients living in a residential care home. They need more help with their 'activities of daily living' such as personal hygiene, going to the toilet, bathing, etc. Some will need to be assisted with their feeding and drinking.

Clients who are admitted to nursing homes need nursing care. In all nursing homes the residents will be suffering from different illnesses and conditions.

A COMPLEX

A complex can either be purpose built or a series of converted buildings.

It is divided into three types of establishment encompassing the three main types of homes. There are a number of warden controlled flats, a residential care home and a nursing home all on the same site.

This means that if your relative starts off in a flat and after a time needs more care, they can be transferred to the part of the complex which will give them the type of care they need. If the illness is a temporary affliction they can return to their flat when they are well again.

Residents do not have to lose their friends when they are moved to a different section of the complex because they are still within walking (or wheelchair) distance of each other.

A complex usually has double rooms for married couples both in the flats and the care home part. There may be some double rooms in the nursing home but the tendency nowadays is to build more single rooms than double rooms.

First component: warden controlled flats

There are a number of flats, some with single bedrooms and others with a double bedroom. Meals can usually be provided but there would probably be an extra charge. Unless a warden is employed the nursing staff visit the flats daily and are on call day and night.

Should the tenant(s) need help they only have to use the internal phone to get assistance. The nursing staff will call the doctor or ambulance if necessary, ie if a person has injured themselves.

Nursing care is not usually provided in the flats but the tenants can be moved into the nursing home if necessary. However the fees will be different to the rent currently paid for the flat.

Second component: residential care home

When the flat becomes too much for the tenant(s) they can move into the care home component provided there is a vacancy. They will receive residential care (see residential care homes page 41) but not nursing care except in an emergency.

Third component: nursing home

If nursing care is needed for any of the tenants or care home residents, nursing staff from the nursing home component will assess the situation. They will take the appropriate action which may entail moving the patient into the nursing wing or sending them by ambulance to the nearest accident and emergency unit.

5

Care Home Facilities

STUDYING THE BROCHURES

Look at the brochures you have received and divide them into three piles:

- instant appeal
- possible
- unsuitable.

Remember:

- Photographs can be misleading; rooms may look more spacious than they are in reality.

- Brochures are a commercial advertisement and can only give you limited information.

- Brochures may be out of date. The home may have new proprietors and/or new managers with new ideas.

Brochures with instant appeal

- Note down what you like about them.

- Do the listed facilities meet your relative's requirements?

- ◆ Look for appropriate homes in the right area.

- ◆ Shortlist the homes that appear to be most suitable.

- ◆ Phone for an appointment to view. Ask for directions if necessary.

- ◆ Note how the phone is answered. Is the person who answered interested, helpful and polite? Their manner might be indicative of the general attitude of the staff.

Avoiding information overload

It's unwise to visit more than three or four homes in a day because:

- ◆ It's exhausting, mentally and physically.

- ◆ It's difficult to remember what you've seen.

- ◆ Absorbing the atmosphere of each home becomes impossible if you have allowed insufficient time.

Before you and your relative can decide, if the home you're currently visiting is the right home for them, you will need to find out as much as you can about the home.

The time to ask all the relevant questions is when you are discussing your relative's needs with the matron. Many people arrive at the matron's office ready to ask the vital questions then find their minds are a complete blank. Most people know what information they need but never think to write down the questions they need to ask. I urge you to take a few minutes and jot down the queries you have.

Some people who have been through the procedure of finding the best nursing or care home for their relative leave the matron's office wishing they had remembered some vital issue they needed to ask about. However, if you do forget to ask something that's a matter of some importance, it's not too late. You can either telephone or make another visit and ask to speak to the person in charge regarding any further queries you have.

THE SIZE OF THE HOME

Some people enjoy being in a home caring for a large number of residents. Others prefer to live and be cared for in smaller ones. There are advantages and disadvantages in both cases.

The larger nursing homes

Larger homes have 50 beds or more. It would be difficult and unusual to have this number of beds plus dining rooms, lounges, toilets and bathrooms, etc all on the ground floor. In view of this there may be two, three or possibly more floors depending on the number of elderly residents they care for.

The residents would be taken to their floor by lift. The largest homes may have two lifts. Access to each floor is also provided by stairways.

In some homes, particularly the more modern ones, the floors are complete with a small kitchen area, lounge and dining area, bathrooms, toilets, nurses' station and treatment room in addition to the bedrooms.

All nursing homes, whether large or small, have communal rooms for the use of residents and their visitors.

Smaller nursing homes

Some homes are designed to be a single storey building, depending on the number of residents they have been built to accommodate.

I have worked in a single storey nursing home built to accommodate 30 residents. There were four wings, three having ten single rooms, each with a second door that opened out onto the garden. Each wing had toilets, bathrooms, linen cupboard, storage space, lounge and dining room in addition to the bedrooms. The fourth wing contained laundry room, offices, storage room and a treatment room. The four wings were arranged around an enclosed circular garden where residents could wander or sit and rest if they wished.

The residents made friends with one another reasonably quickly and enjoyed any activities the staff arranged for them, particularly at Christmas.

Although it is perhaps easier for the residents to make new friends in smaller homes, it can be just as easy in the larger homes. They can ask to sit in a particular group with their new friends and join in activities if they wish. It is possible that there will be a wider range of activities in the larger homes because the higher the number of residents the wider the range of interests which need to be catered for.

ROOM SIZES AND SUITABILITY

The modern trend is for nursing and residential care homes to have single rooms only but there are some which have a combination of single and double rooms. Double rooms are often used for married couples but not always. All double rooms should have curtains or a screen to divide the room when one or both residents need privacy.

The size of the rooms varies according to the needs of the kind of residents the home is registered to care for and whether the rooms are to be used as single or double rooms. The Inspecting Officers will advise the home owner if any of the rooms designated as a resident's room does not conform to the regulations and is therefore unsuitable for that purpose.

Warden controlled flats are variable in size, some are built for single people whilst others cater for married couples.

In new building projects regulations state that rooms must be of a certain size. Nursing home rooms have to be larger than in residential care homes. This is to enable staff to bring hoists, dressing trolleys, special beds or other equipment into the room when necessary.

When large houses are converted into nursing or care homes the rooms are measured and designated for either nursing or residential care. If the proprietor wishes to accommodate both kinds of residents they will need to apply for dual registration which, if granted, will allow them to use the rooms as designated, providing their levels of trained nursing staff and care assistants comply with the regulations.

When making their inspection of the bedrooms Inspectors will take into consideration:

◆ room size

◆ decor

◆ windows

◆ door size and wheelchair access

◆ furniture

◆ safety such as: very hot water from the hot water tap; wrinkled carpets, ruckled linoleum or rugs which could cause a resident to trip, etc

◆ unshielded radiators

◆ general suitability.

En suite facilities

Not all homes have en suite rooms. Some establishments have rooms with their own bathroom facilities, others only have a toilet. All rooms are provided with a hand basin and hot and cold water.

En suite facilities are often too small to be of use to an elderly disabled person. Unless your relative can do most things for themselves they may find it easier to use the communal bathrooms and toilets where there is more space and bathing equipment, making it safer and easier for them.

FACILITIES

Laundry services

Almost all homes have an in-house laundry where residents' clothing is washed and ironed and taken back to the person's room and put away. Unfortunately if clothing is not marked with the resident's name it can get mislaid.

Laundry services do not generally include articles that need to be dry-cleaned and it is usually the responsibility of the resident's relatives to take the clothes to the dry cleaners and pay for this service themselves. If the home agrees to take clothing that needs dry-cleaning to the appropriate place to be dealt with, there will be an extra charge to cover the cost of this service.

GP services

Your relative's current doctor may be willing to continue to visit, monitor their progress, advise, and prescribe for them if and when they succumb to illness, on condition the surgery is near the home.

However, if it is not practical for your relative's own doctor to continue caring for them, they will have the opportunity to change to a more local practice. The matron will advise in this case.

Sometimes patients are not very happy with the treatment they receive from their current GP and would be pleased to be transferred to another doctor's list at this time.

Most doctors arrange for their patients, in all types of residential care, to receive their annual flu vaccination as a preventative measure, providing they are willing to take advantage of it.

Activities

Many care establishments have an activities programme. Some employ a person to draw up a daily activities list and put it into operation. It is difficult to suit all the residents all the time. They may enjoy some activities more than others but if they join in they will make new friends and enrich their lives.

The activities might include such things as craft work; story telling; games; bingo; cards; music and movement;* board games; listening to audio tapes; video tapes, making items for special functions such as Christmas; knitting or sewing. Some care establishments are fortunate enough to own a mini-bus which they use to take the residents to the local town or places of interest.

If your relative has a particular hobby ask the matron if it can be included in the activities.

---

*Although music and movement is a very gentle exercise programme your relative's doctor should be asked if their patient is fit enough to participate, particularly if they have a pacemaker.

Entertainment

On occasions there may be a solo musician or group who will visit and entertain the residents. The matron would have to make arrangements with such a person or company if the fee does not exceed the amount budgeted for entertainments. The artistes are not always well known but they bring a smile and an interest to the residents, especially if they sing the popular songs of the residents' youth. Sometimes the staff will band together and put on a concert themselves for the residents and their visitors.

Library services

There is generally a library within the homes for those residents who like to read. Sometimes the books are donated but in some areas the local library is able to bring a selection of books initially and change them at regular intervals. If there is no such facility, books can be borrowed by friends or relatives on a resident's behalf from the local library. However, the person borrowing the books is generally responsible for their safe return at the proper time. Secondhand books can also be purchased from charity shops, boot fairs, jumble sales or market stalls.

Trolley shop

There are always a few residents who are too disabled or who have no inclination to go out. In nursing homes the residents are often too sick or frail to even think of leaving the home. With this in mind some matrons organise a weekly shopping trolley with things such as writing paper, envelopes, stamps and other useful items that the residents can purchase.

Gardens

Many homes have lovely gardens for the residents to rest or walk in. Sometimes the home's gardener or handyman will help residents to plant hanging baskets or tubs or even bulbs for them to have in their rooms or communal areas. It may even be possible to have raised flower beds to enable keen gardeners, if they are fit and well enough, to enjoy gardening again.

Religious services

The matron may already have arranged to have church services held within the home by the local clergy or pastors. If there is no religious service suitable for your relative, bring the matter up with the matron. They may be able to contact the appropriate minister and ask them to visit your relative when admitted. Alternatively, depending on distance, you could ask their own minister to visit.

Car parking

Many of the residents' visitors will have their own transport. One of their biggest worries is where they can park the car.

Most homes outside a city or town have car parking facilities both for staff and visitors. It is sometimes more difficult if the home is situated on a busy road with little or no space to park a car. The matron or the staff will know where the nearest parking places are. If the home is fortunate enough to have a car park it may prove difficult to find. When you phone to make an appointment to view the home, ask how to find it.

Christmas

Many residents go out on Christmas Day to relatives or friends, some go and stay over the whole of the Christmas period. However, many remain in the home.

Christmas is a happy time almost everywhere, care and nursing homes are no exception. The extent of the festivities depends on the proprietor, matron and all other staff. Staff generally put up decorations a few days beforehand. A Christmas tree arrives and is dressed with lights and tinsel. The chef makes mince pies and all the other goodies that make Christmas so happy.

Many organisations go round the homes singing carols, bringing their own brand of cheerfulness and happiness. It is not unknown for Father Christmas to make an appearance on Christmas morning or at some other time during the Christmas season. Everywhere is decorated with cards and wrapped parcels. Christmas lunch is served and enjoyed. The afternoon is for visitors, watching the television, games or snoozing. I have never known anybody not enjoy Christmas in a home unless they are too ill.

Residents' visitors

Visitors are encouraged to join in the fun but if they wish to have lunch with their relative, arrangements need to be made with the matron a few days in advance.

Taking gifts

Please make sure gifts are marked with your relative's name otherwise they may go astray because nobody will know to whom they belong.

6

Gathering Information

FINDING OUT WHERE CARE HOMES ARE LOCATED

You can live in an area for years and not realise there are nursing or residential care homes nearby. You can find out about them as follows.

◆ Contact your nearest Social Services' Care Line and ask advice. They will send you all the information you need including a list of all types of homes in the area and tell you who to contact if the information you need is dealt with in another department. A care manager will advise you on the correct procedure to take if your relative wishes to be placed in a home in another town to be near you, their friends, or other members of the family.

◆ Look in your local telephone book to see care home advertisements.

◆ Your doctor's surgery may also be able to help.

Involving a care manager

Care managers are not allowed to recommend any particular care home. You have to investigate the most suitable homes for yourself. However, a care manager will visit your relative and assess their needs and tell you which type of home is most suitable for your relative. A care manager will be able to give advice regarding the financial problems associated with transferring your relative into a residential care home or nursing home. Initially they will discuss the financial situation with you themselves but ultimately will refer your relative to their finance department which will arrange for them to have a financial assessment carried out if necessary. A financial assessment has to be done before any funding can be granted.

Once your relative has been place in a suitable home the care manager will visit them after a few weeks to review the situation and make changes if necessary. Nursing staff, the next of kin and the resident are usually invited to such a meeting so that they can talk about present or potential problems and how they might be resolved.

There is, of course, no need to involve a care manager if your relative's assets are in excess of the figure where they can obtain financial help, currently £19,500. This figure is subject to change on an annual basis. The care manager or the finance officer will be able to give you the current figure.

Personal recommendations

One of the best ways to find out about a care home is to ask somebody who already has a relative or friend living in such a place. People are always ready to give inside information if you ask them. They may even invite you to visit their friend or relation with them.

You must be careful to ensure that it is the type of care home your relative needs. Remember, even if the home appears to be the perfect place for your friend's relative it may not be the perfect place for your relative.

Brochures
Once you have decided which homes you and your relative are interested in telephone the matron or manager and ask them to send brochures and further information, such as a list of fees and extras, if any.

Location
Once you know for sure which type of home you are looking for you can see from the list you have made which nursing or residential care homes appear to be most suitable regarding access.

If you have a car it is easier to drive round and see the location of the various homes. Any that would be difficult to get to if you had no means of visiting without your own transport should not really be considered unless public transport to or near the home is reliable and fairly frequent. Remember their friends and possibly other members of the family will be in the same age group, and may be unable to drive but still want to visit your relative.

VISITING HOMES
Having decided which homes appear to be most suitable make an appointment to view. Compile a list of things you want to see and ask. Take the list with you. It is much easier to remember to ask what you really want to know if it's written down (see Figure 1).

What to see and ask	Home 1 The Willows comments
Access to rooms	
Activites	
Are there any extras to pay for?	
Bath hoists	
Bathrooms and special baths	
Bedrooms	
Commode	
Dining room	
En suite	
Furniture	
Gardens	
General hoists	
Insurance certificate	
Kitchens	
Lifts	
Lounge	
Meal times	
Menus	
Pets	
Position of toilets	
Post	
Quiet room	
Registration Certificate	
Residents' charter	
Smokers' room	
Staffing levels – day and night	
What's included in the fees	
Wheelchair ramps	

Fig. 1. Checklist 1.

The matron or a senior member of staff will show you the layout of the home, the residents' rooms, communal rooms, bathrooms, etc.

You will see different aspects of nursing home life, depending on which time of the day you visit. If you visit at lunch time you may be able to visit the dining room, look at and smell the food. Is it appetising? Are the residents enjoying their meal? Do they look happy? Do they respond when you speak to them?

If you make an afternoon visit you may see a number of the residents enjoying some form of planned activity or entertainment; others might be resting or watching television.

Draw up a chart showing the things you notice in each home (Figure 1). If you jot them down at each visit you will not forget what you have seen. When you enter them on to a master chart differences between the homes you visit will become much more apparent (see Figure 2).

Planning your visit

Shortlist a few homes (about three: see Figure 3) you think would be most suitable for your relative. If you don't see the matron on your first visit to the two or three preferred homes, you should make an appointment to see them on your second visit.

They will need to know all about your relative. This is why you need the written details you prepared when you assessed your relative's needs (Chapter 1 Assessing your relative's needs).

What to see and ask	Home 1	Home 2	Home 3
Access to rooms			
Activites			
Are there any extras to pay for?			
Bath hoists			
Bathrooms and special baths			
Bedrooms			
Commode			
Dining room			
En suite			
Furniture			
Gardens			
General hoists			
Insurance certificate			
Kitchens			
Lifts			
Lounge			
Meal times			
Menus			
Pets			
Position of toilets			
Post			
Quiet room			
Registration Certificate			
Residents' charter			
Smokers' room			
Staffing levels – day and night			
What's included in the fees			
Wheelchair ramps			

Fig. 2. Comparison chart first visit.

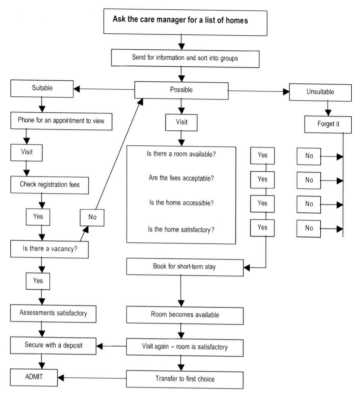

Fig. 3. Sorting the information.

You might like to ask questions, such as:

1. Can my Mum have a single room?

2. My relative is a diabetic, will a diabetic diet be provided?

3. My Aunt is incontinent of urine, will pads be provided?

4. Are incontinent pads, etc included in the fees or is there a charge?

5. If there is a charge, how much will it cost per calendar month?

6. Is there an in-house laundry for residents' personal clothing?

7. Is there an extra charge for this? If so, how much will it cost?

8. Is there insurance cover for clothing lost or damaged during laundering?

9. My Dad weighs about 16 stone (100kg) Will he be able to have a bath?

10. My Grandma is a Christian, can she go to church if somebody comes and fetches her? What about her meals in this case?

11. My relative is of the RC, Jewish, Muslim or other faith, will they be able to receive spiritual help?

12. Are there any provisions for in-house church services?

13. Does my Mum's own doctor visit this home?

14. What are the visiting hours?

15. What are the fees? Are there any extras to be met?

16. Some of my aunt's visitors live several miles away, can they have lunch?

17. Can visitors have a cup of tea or coffee during their visit?

18. How do I make a complaint?

19. To what extent are the residents involved when there is a fire drill?

20. What happens if my Dad falls and sustains a fracture and needs to go to hospital?

21. Is there a visiting hairdresser?

22. What kind of activities are provided for the residents?

23. Are the residents ever taken out by the staff?

24. Does the home have any functions, such as fetes, parties, Christmas?

25. My Aunt has a leg ulcer. Can that be attended to here?

26. Granny doesn't like to breathe in cigarette smoke. Is there a no smoking policy here? Or, my relative likes to smoke occasionally, is that allowed?

27. My aunt likes to have a small glass of sherry about eight o'clock. Would that be a problem?

28. Dad takes several prescribed tablets and medicines plus vitamins and minerals. How will he obtain them or will they be given to him at the appropriate times?

29. Mum doesn't always sleep very well. It helps her to have a cup of tea in the night. Would that be possible?

30. Are there any rules that we need to be aware of?

The above questions are a few of the queries anxious relatives or prospective residents ask. You will probably think of other queries which are applicable to your relative.

Speaking to staff

If possible have a chat to some of the staff while you're making your visit. Note their attitude, whether they are happy. Happy staff tend to make happy residents!

Using your five senses

Smell

This sense comes into play as soon as the door is opened to you.

- Does the home smell clean?

- Is there an odour of urine as you enter?

- Is there a smell of body odour?

- Do the toilets and bathrooms smell sweet?

- Are there any smells of stale food or cooking hanging around?

Touch

The things you touch should feel clean, particularly in the dining room.

- Are the chairs clean and dry?

- Is furniture that should be polished, polished or needing attention?

Sight

What do you see?

- Are the residents looking clean and well cared for? If a resident has spilled something, it will obviously take a few minutes for it to be noticed and their clothing changed.

- Do the residents look happy and comfortable?

- Are the staff wearing clean uniforms or clean personal clothing?

Hearing
What do you hear?

- Do you hear the sound of laughter? Talking? Pleasant or not so pleasant?

- Do you hear residents talking to each other, or is it staff talking to each other – ignoring the residents?

- Is the television on full blast drowning out everything else?

Taste
You may not get a chance to use this sense. Assuming that you are given a cup of tea or coffee and a biscuit or piece of cake take time to taste whether your drink is really hot or lukewarm, whether the milk is fresh or on the turn.

- Is the cake or biscuit fresh or stale?

This will give a small indication of how food is used and presented to the residents.

RULES

There are usually a few rules that need to be adhered to for the safety of the home and residents. They are generally kept to a minimum but might include:

◆ keeping fire doors closed;

◆ keeping fire exit doors free from obstruction i.e. cases or wheelchairs;

◆ medications being locked away;

◆ medications being taken under supervision;

◆ hoists being used for residents over a certain weight;

◆ residents being barred from certain areas, eg kitchens, laundry, etc.

INSPECTIONS AND CERTIFICATES

All residential and nursing homes for the elderly are inspected regularly on a number of points. This is to ensure:

◆ the premises are safe and clean;

◆ the residents are clean, comfortable and happy;

◆ the kitchens and foodstuffs are stored properly, safe and clean;

◆ menus are balanced, enjoyable and have choice;

◆ all drugs (medications) are properly stored, dispensed and recorded;

◆ care of individual residents is carried out properly and well;

♦ that all care, allergies, treatment and other important information is recorded correctly.

There are many other things that are inspected over and above these listed items.

National Care Standard Commission

These inspections are carried out by the National Care Standard Commission. Sometimes the home is notified of an impending inspection in order that the person in charge can get all the books, certificates, residents' care plans, fire and maintenance records, kitchen records and menus, etc ready for the inspectors to see. The inspectors leave or send a report to be kept in the home. You are at liberty to ask to see these reports if you so wish.

The fire service

Fire officers also make visits to check fire exits are free, there are no fire hazards resulting from excess rubbish within the home and to look for anything else which is a potential fire hazard. They check fire and smoke alarms, fire hoses, fire-blankets (kitchen) and the fire zone alarm system.

All residential homes have to test fire alarms on a regular basis. If any fail to function they have to be dealt with. The fault, the date and time of repair and times and dates of testing must be recorded. The fire officer will check all records of fire equipment and staff training each time they come.

District pharmacist

Another inspection which takes place is in the treatment room where the medicine trolley is kept. All the medications (drugs), ointments, creams, injections, controlled drugs and records are checked by the district pharmacist regularly.

These three inspections are the main ones. Each inspection helps to ensure the well-being of the residents.

Residents' charter

Most homes have a residents' charter. Sometimes this is on display. If you wish to see it or have a copy ask the matron or the nurse in charge (see sample in Figure 4).

Registration and insurance certificates

These certificates should be on display for visitors to see. They are usually framed and hanging on a wall in the reception area of the home. If you cannot find them ask the matron or the nurse in charge to show you where they are.

CHECKLIST

Have you looked through the brochures and discussed them with your relative?

◆ Have you made a list of the questions you want to ask?

◆ Have you made a list of the things you wish to see?

Residents' Charter of Rights

Introduction

It is the policy of the home to provide quality personal care and to recognise the rights of the individual to: privacy; dignity; independence; freedom of choice and the right to have as much control over their life as possible.

Charter of rights

As a resident you have the right to:

Bring into the home any possessions and/or small items of furniture provided the furniture is sound, free of wood-worm and is within the confines of the space available in your allotted room.

Choose how and with whom you spend your day.

Have access to your own room when you wish.

Entertain any visitors in your room and invite people to visit you when you wish.

Get up and go to bed when you please.

Manage your own finances.

Take part in any social or recreational activities, organised by the staff within the home, of your choosing.

Have access to any written material directly concerning you held by the management.

Have the right to expect that any information imparted to a member of staff will be treated with respect and confidentiality.

Be involved in any discussions about your care.

Take part in any religious services arranged in the home and to attend your own place of worship.

Select your meals from the menu and eat when you wish.

Choose your own bathing times.

Wear your own clothes as you wish.

Help in the running of the home by attending the monthly management and residents' committee meetings.

Have access to your care manager and social services department.

Have access to a doctor, dentist, physiotherapist, optician and solicitor.

Be able to complain without fear of reprisal.

Be called by the name of your choice.

Have the right to expect the staff to arrange transport to any booked hospital appointments within the limits of the service.

Fig. 4. Sample Residents' Charter.

(7)

Finances

INVOLVING SOCIAL SERVICES

Whilst it is not obligatory to involve Social Services, particularly if your relative is going to be self-funding (being totally responsible for their own fees) it is best to inform them and ask for advice as soon as you or your doctor realise your relative needs full-time care.

A care manager will be appointed to help and advise. They will:

- Make an assessment regarding the most appropriate type of care required.

- Arrange a financial assessment if required.

- Give you a comprehensive list of homes in the area.

- Inform you which homes will give the type of care your relative needs.

- Arrange respite care during the waiting period if necessary.

- Reassess the placement of your relative during the first few weeks.

- Advise you if the placement is unsuitable and help find a more appropriate home for your relative.

If Social Services is involved four assessments will be made:

1. Assessment by a care manager to establish the type of care required.

2. A financial assessment to determine your relative's contribution towards care.

3. An assessment by the matron of the care home to establish whether the chosen home is the best possible home for your relative.

4. An assessment by the health authority to determine if your relative requires nursing care. If they do it will be decided how much nursing care need.

If Social Services are not involved only assessments 3 and 4 will apply.

The reason for the last assessment to determine the amount of nursing care a resident will need is because the National Health Service now pays for nursing services within nursing homes. This means that the resident no longer has to pay for this component of their care.

COMPARING FEES

All homes have their own fee structure. Most homes charge different rates for single rooms, double rooms and for en suite facilities. Some homes will only admit residents who are self-funding, others will also admit those who are being helped by Social Services; some homes only admit residents who rely on Social Services for their funding.

It is sensible to contact your local Social Services offices and ask for a financial assessment before making any final decisions regarding your relative's transfer to a care home.

Your relative's care manager will assess the needs of your relative and decide the type of care which is most appropriate for them. This may be a residential care home, a nursing home or another type of care. If you disagree with their decision you may ask for a second opinion.

They will give you a list of homes in the area and guidance regarding the listed homes which may be suitable for your relative. However, care managers are not allowed to recommend any particular home.

Before you visit the various homes jot down a list of financial issues you need to know about, for instance:

- Will a monthly account be sent to me?

- Do the fees cover everything?

- Are there any extra charges for anything?

- When are fees due?

- Can fees be paid by direct debit?

- Who are the direct debit or cheques made payable to?

- Do Social Services send their contribution to the home?

Your care manager will arrange for your relative to have a financial assessment. This is mandatory if they hope to have financial help from Social Services. Even those people who expect to be self-funding may benefit from such an assessment because the assessor will ensure your relative is getting all the allowances to which they are entitled.

THE FINANCIAL ASSESSMENT

An appointment will be made for a financial assessment to be carried out by one of the staff of the financial department of Social Services. They will visit your relative, provided they wish to have such an assessment which your relative is at liberty to refuse. You will be able to be with them during the assessment.

The assessor will need to know the source of your relative's total income including any regular amounts of money from grants.

Some examples of income that the finance officer will need details of:

♦ State pension.

♦ Other pensions including disability; invalidity; industrial and war pensions.

♦ All allowances including attendance and disability living allowance.

♦ Net earnings and sick pay.

♦ Income from tenants and non-dependent relatives.

♦ Annuities and all other income.

Some other sources of income

Your relative may have monthly or quarterly income from:

- investments

- savings

- stocks and shares

- rented property

- seasonal lettings from holiday homes or caravans, etc

- full- or part-time work

- working from home

- charitable grants.

At the time of writing:

- If your relative has savings and investments of over £19,500 they will have to pay the full cost of care. In this case they will not have to divulge any information regarding their income.

- If your relative has savings and investments between £12,000 and £19,499 they may have to contribute something from their savings towards the cost of care.

- If they have less than £12,000 nothing will be taken from their investments or savings.

- Bear in mind that pensions, allowances, residents' contributions toward their care, etc are subject to change annually or even more frequently. Check them with your care manager or Social Services finance department (see Figure 5).

Your relative's house

If your relative owns their own home and leaves it to enter into a care home permanently the house will be counted as an asset after the first 12 weeks. If their spouse or one of their relatives continues to live there it may not

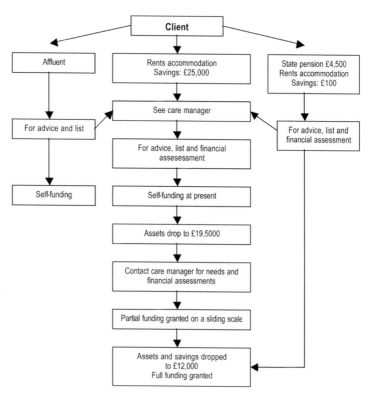

Fig. 5. Qualifying for funding.

be taken into account. However, if they own more than one property the second house will be taken into consideration.

Although this information is accurate for East Sussex it is possible that there may be minor changes in different counties of England.

Wherever your relative lives it would be wise to telephone or write to your local Social Services office and ask for information. They will send you a variety of helpful booklets with useful addresses and telephone numbers of relevant organisations.

BASIC FEES

Sometimes the home's basic fees are listed on the brochure but not always.

You may be given a list of fees (see Figure 6) or they may be discussed when you go to view the home and see the matron. You should ask if there are any items for which you are expected to pay extra.

Generally speaking the basic fee includes:

◆ care

◆ the resident's room

◆ bed linen

◆ towels

◆ meals including elevenses, afternoon tea and night drinks, etc

---

HIGHFIELD NURSING HOME

List of fees

Facility	Daily fee	Weekly fee	Monthly fee*
Shared room per person	£69.00	£483.00	£2,093.00
Shared room with en suite per person	£71.00	£497.00	£2,153.00
Single room	£73.00	£511.00	£2,214.33
Single room with en suite	£75.00	£525.00	£2,275.00
Double room used as a single	£123.50	£864.50	£3,746.17
Short-term rates: (less than one calendar month)	75.00 per person per day		
Absences (hospitalisation or holidays, etc)			
Less than seven days	No reduction		
More than seven days	10% reduction		
*Monthly fee means calendar month			

Fig. 6. Sample fees list.

♦ laundering of machine washable personal clothing

♦ light and heating.

Items which may attract extra charges in some homes
All homes are different and what is included in the fees of one home may be classed as an extra in another, such as:

♦ double rooms used as a single room

♦ en suite facilities

♦ refreshments and meals for visitors

♦ incontinence aids

♦ hiring of special equipment

♦ heavily dependent residents

- extra staff for one-to-one basis in special circumstances

- personal laundry and dry cleaning

- occupational therapy materials

- hairdressing

- outings

- speech therapy

- chiropody

- private consultants' and doctors' visits

- private prescriptions

- shopping

- anything else the management considers is not covered by the basic fee.

Find out what is included and what is termed an extra.

PAYING THE ACCOUNTS

The matron will probably suggest that the fees are paid by direct debit and will give you the appropriate form if you wish. This will ensure that the money is debited form your relative's bank account and transferred into the home's account on the due date.

Providing the home manager is in agreement the fees can be paid by cheque on or before the due date.

It is very unusual for residents or their relatives to pay with cash and in this case the proprietor and the manager must be in agreement in allowing this method of payment as special arrangements would have to be made to receive such substantial amounts of cash.

APPLYING FOR A GRANT

It may have been suggested that your relative should apply for a grant from a charitable organisation. There are many charities that may offer financial support either by a one-off payment, perhaps for clothing or a piece of equipment such as a type of computer to aid speech or mobility aids.

Finding charities that may offer help

◆ Set aside a morning or afternoon to do some research armed with an A4 notepad and biros.

◆ Go to the reference section in the main library in your area.

◆ Ask the librarian for *The Encyclopaedia of Charities UK 2003 Edition 15*. This book has 31 sections and 8,000 listed charities.

◆ Read through the index of each section which might be suitable for your relative's needs and write down the numbers, eg Diabetes 426; Stroke Association 438; this will help you find them more easily without having to keep referring to the index.

◆ Check each entry to discover whether your relative might qualify for a grant.

◆ Jot down the name of all the organisations which you think might offer help. Make a note of each organisation's name, address, telephone number and person to contact if it is given.

♦ Take the details of as many as you can including what they appear to be offering.

The next step
♦ Study the list at home.

♦ Phone the organisation and check the name of the person to whom you should apply.

♦ Write a letter stating your relative's circumstances and needs to the three most likely organisations (see Figure 7).

♦ They will probably send you a formal application form. Fill it in accurately, black biro is best, sign and return it with any required documentation to support the application as soon as possible.

♦ Keep copies of all correspondence for your reference.

♦ Wait patiently for their reply.

♦ If the first three cannot help write to the next three and so on.

♦ Letters asking for financial assistance usually have to be discussed at a committee meeting and it may take some weeks before you receive an answer.

You will find various organisations only apply to a certain group of people, for instance some charities only consider people born and bred in a certain place. If your relative does not fulfil the criteria don't apply.

Do remember that any grant your relative receives must be declared at their financial assessment.

Ashcroft
28 Any Street
Nonsuch Town
XY0 Z01

Mrs G Goldsmith, Director
Appropriate Charitable Society
Bentley House
Rolls Road
Any Town BX0 0XB

Mrs Goldsmith,
I am writing on behalf of my friend who needs money for some new winter clothing.

Her name is Mrs Annie Drew born in Anytown on 24th May 1925.

She left school when she was 15 years of age and worked as a children's nanny until she married at the age of 35. She has never been in pensionable employment.

Since her marriage she has cared for her son, now age 30, who has learning difficulties. A few years ago her husband lost his sight in a road accident and has since developed carcinoma of the bowel for which he has undergone surgery. He is now very frail.

Annie is still in hospital recovering from a heart attack but she is almost ready to be discharged. Fred her husband has also been admitted as he needs more treatment and constant care. Kevin, their son has been admitted to Sunshine House for a few weeks. The couple have no relatives.

Annie and Fred are being transferred to the nursing wing in the Devonshire Complex as soon as Annie is considered fit enough.

Annie has no suitable clothing to take with her although what she has is clean well patched, and darned, but is threadbare and has no warmth left in it.

There has been little money coming into the home during the last few years and what money there was has been spent on essentials such as food and heating. Any money left over has been spent on their son's needs.

I would be grateful if you could offer some assistance in order that Annie can have some warm clothing for the coming winter months.

Yours sincerely,

Elizabeth Green

Fig. 7. Sample grants application letter.

SARAH'S STORY

Sarah lived alone after the sudden death of her husband, Keith, in 1998. Keith had always kept the garden looking lovely and Sarah had always kept the bungalow in a pristine condition. Now, after four long years, she was struggling. The garden was too much for her, the steps to the front and back doors were steep and difficult.

She decided to sell the bungalow and move into a care home. Her nephew suggested she went to live in the Bournemouth area, near some of the family.

'After all,' he said, 'your sister lives in Penny Lodge Nursing Home, why don't you live there?'

He took Sarah to the nursing home to see her sister who was very sick indeed. The proprietor knew the circumstances and offered Sarah a lovely room on the ground floor which she accepted and put down a deposit. Sarah was fine until she was back in her own home again, then she realised she would be living in Bournemouth and all her friends would be living in Eastbourne.

Then the tears flowed, Sarah became more and more depressed.

'Why don't you stay up here where all your friends are?' I asked her one day.

'Because my sister is ill and I ought to be there with her.'

'What will you do if your sister doesn't get better?'

'I don't know, she has her own room and she can't speak very much now, she's too ill.'

Several people suggested she stayed in the area where she knew so many people.

One day she told me she had changed her mind about going to live in Bournemouth. 'The only thing is, I've got nowhere to live now and the house sale is going through. We exchange contracts in a couple of weeks.' Sarah thought of one of our mutual friends who lives in a warden controlled flat.

She phoned and asked if there were any flats vacant. There was and Sarah made an appointment to view. In the meantime she met somebody else who told her about a beautiful residential home in Eastbourne. She liked the sound of it. She cancelled the appointment to view the flat.

'I'm going to live at Birchwood Manor' Sarah told me the next time I saw her.

'I thought you were going to live in a warden controlled flat near Elsie.'

'Oh, I've changed my mind. I don't want to cook any more.' she explained.

'Anyway, I've seen the room I'm going to have, it's spacious and on the top floor. There's a shower and toilet and a sort of mini kitchen. I think I shall be happy there.'

'When are you moving in?'

'Next Wednesday,' Sarah replied. 'You will come and see me won't you?'

A few weeks later I visited Sarah in her new home and admired her choice. She seemed to be quite comfortable and happy.

Because her assets were above £19,500 she didn't need to contact Social Services.

(8)

Food and Drink

MEAL TIMES

All homes set their meal times for the benefit of the residents. Because of this meal times vary from home to home. Generally speaking breakfast is usually served between 8 and 9am. Lunch between 12.30 and 1pm and 'high tea' or dinner between 5 and 6.30pm.

Coffee, tea or other drinks and a biscuit are served about 10.30–11am and afternoon tea about 3pm.

Night drinks such as hot chocolate, horlicks, tea, milk, etc are usually brought round by the night nurses about 8.30–9.30pm. If a resident wants a hot drink during the night hours they only have to ring the call bell and a member of staff will make one for them.

Where are meals served?

In some homes, particularly residential care homes, breakfast is served in the dining area but in other homes it is served in residents' rooms.

In homes where breakfast is served in the dining room residents can usually choose where they prefer to eat the first meal of the day, either in their rooms or in the dining area, depending on the their health.

Lunch and high tea (or dinner) are usually served in the dining room or the dining area of the lounge for those residents who are able to be brought to the table.

For residents who are sick meals are served to them in their rooms.

Some residents prefer to have all their meals served in the lounge, others wish to remain in their room all the time including meals times. Whilst this is not forbidden it is generally discouraged, because the resident:

◆ doesn't get the chance to make friends

◆ tends to withdraw from activities because they don't know other residents

◆ can become introverted

◆ can become isolated

◆ can become depressed.

Elevenses and afternoon tea are served to the residents wherever they happen to be in the home at the time (except the bathroom or toilet).

A community spirit, friendship and chatting between the residents is encouraged particularly at meal times.

Eating a meal

Some residents are physically incapable of feeding themselves and will be fed, or helped to feed themselves, by care staff.

Blind residents are helped if the food is served onto their plate in a pattern, such as a clock. The resident is asked to imagine the plate as if it were a clock. Potatoes might be served on the plate at the 12 o'clock position; meat/fish served on the plate at the 6 o'clock position; the first vegetable, eg broccoli might be placed on the plate at 3 o'clock position, the second vegetable, eg carrots, at the 9 o'clock position, sauces or condiments at the 7 o'clock position.

If the blind resident is told clearly and understands where the different foods, eg vegetables or meat have been placed (in relation to a clock face numerals) they will probably be able to feed themselves with little or no help within a short period of time. See Figure 8.

MENUS

Part of the chef's job is to ensure meals are nutritious, well balanced, well cooked and served attractively.

Meals are not produced haphazardly but with thought and planning. A series of weekly menus are drawn up and numbered one to four or six by the chef to cover a period of four or six weeks At the end of that period it is repeated starting again at week one.

The menu sets out what is planned for breakfast, lunch and high tea or dinner each day, plus an alternative dish for each meal.

New menus are usually drawn up every season in order that residents may have the benefit of seasonal fruits and

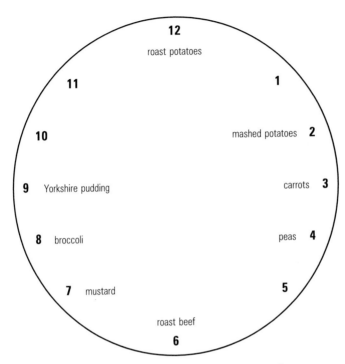

Fig. 8. Food on a plate relating to clock numerals.

vegetables. The expected seasonal weather is also taken into consideration. In winter you get more winter foods like stew and dumplings and steamed puddings on the menu. The summer menu will offer more salads and cold sweets.

Although the menus are set, alternatives can always be offered particularly on days that are not so seasonal. See sample menu Figure 9.

Alternative choices

All homes should always be able to offer alternatives even if they are not listed on the menu due to lack of space.

	Monday	Tuesday	Wednesday	Thursday	Friday	Saturday	Sunday
Breakfast	Fruit juice Fresh fruit Porridge Choice of cereals Toast and preserves Tea or coffee	Fruit juice Fresh fruit Porridge Choice of cereals Toast and preserves Tea or coffee	Fruit juice Fresh fruit Porridge Choice of cereals Toast and preserves Tea or coffee	Fruit juice Fresh fruit Porridge Choice of cereals Toast and preserves Tea or coffee	Fruit juice Fresh fruit Porridge Choice of cereals Toast and preserves Tea or coffee	Fruit juice Fresh fruit Porridge Choice of cereals Toast and preserves Tea or coffee	Fruit juice Fresh fruit Porridge Choice of cereals Toast and preserves Tea or coffee
Lunch	Shepherd's pie Boiled potatoes Seasonal vegetables *Dessert* Ginger sponge and custard Cheese and biscuits	Chicken casserole Creamed potatoes Broccoli *Dessert* Apple pie and custard Cheese and biscuits	Roast pork Boiled potatoes Seasonal vegetables *Dessert* Rice pudding or ice cream Cheese and biscuits	Lamb stew Potato pie Seasonal vegetables *Dessert* Rhubarb crumble and custard Cheese and biscuits	Fried fish and chips or Poached fish Creamed potatoes *Dessert* Stewed apricots and custard Cheese and biscuits	Gammon steak Parsley sauce Creamed or boiled potatoes and peas *Dessert* Pineapple-upside-down-cake and custard Cheese and biscuits	Roast chicken Roast potatoes Seasonal vegetables stuffing, gravy *Dessert* Fruit salad and cream Cheese and biscuits
Dinner	Soup Macaroni cheese Assorted sandwiches *Dessert* Yoghurt	Soup Fish cakes Assorted sandwiches *Dessert* Banana mousse	Soup Cornish pasties Assorted sandwiches *Dessert* Fruit jelly	Soup Chicken nuggets Assorted sandwiches *Dessert* Creme caramel	Soup Lasagne Assorted sandwiches *Dessert* Semolina and jam	Soup Corned beef hash Assorted sandwiches *Dessert* Fruit cake	Soup Scrambled egg on toast Assorted sandwiches *Dessert* Profiteroles

Water or Squash is served with lunch and dinner. Tea or coffee is served after lunch and dinner.
Alternative dishes, ice cream, cheese and biscuits are always available if required.

Fig. 9. Sample of a weekly menu.

When you're looking at the various establishments ask the matron if you can see the current menu and if alternative choices are not listed, ask if a choice is provided if a meal is unsuitable in any way for your relative.

Likes and dislikes
Most of us dislike certain foods or flavours. If there is anything on the menu which your relative dislikes they can ask the staff for an alternative dish.

MEALS AND REFRESHMENTS FOR VISITORS
Most homes will offer visitors a cup of tea or coffee if they are with their relative at the appropriate time. This is usually free of charge but if you ask for a tray of tea or coffee a charge may be made.

If you wish to have a meal with your relative you would need to ask as soon as you arrive or preferably by phone the day before. In some homes they do not charge for the meal but others add a charge to the resident's account.

It makes sense to keep a record of all meals and refreshments you are given in case a mistake is made and you are charged for something you have not had.

SWEETS, CHOCOLATE AND BISCUITS
Biscuits usually accompany morning and afternoon tea or coffee but you are generally allowed to take in extra biscuits as well as sweets, chocolate, fruit, squash, etc for the resident to keep in their room. Before you do, check with staff regarding your relative's diet and if there are any restrictions on what you may take in for them.

It's a good idea to take in a fruit bowl and suitable receptacles for sweets and biscuits marked with your relative's name to keep their goodies in.

SPECIAL DIETS

Special diets are ordered by doctors or consultants for people with certain medical complaints. These people need a diet that will do them no harm and will enable them, in most cases, to live a reasonably normal life. For instance, residents suffering from diabetes need a diet which maintains the balance of their blood sugar and insulin levels. This particular diet is one where the person can maintain the correct sugar intake by an exchange system rather than a set daily menu. Leaflets explaining this system are usually found at the diabetic clinic or the doctor's surgery.

Other residents may need a low fat or low salt diet to prevent deterioration.

Allergies

Your relative may be a person who suffers from one or more food allergies. Common causes of allergies are strawberries and shellfish but dairy foods and nuts as well as many other foods can produce an allergic reaction. For some, peanuts or anything containing peanuts or even a smear of peanut oil is lethal.

Residents with any kind of food allergy must have a diet which excludes the foods or ingredients which cause the problem.

The chef will be well aware of diets and allergies and will produce any special diets required by residents who need them for their well being.

Please inform the matron of any:

◆ special diets

◆ allergies to certain foods

◆ allergy to any medications, wasp, bee or other insect stings

◆ allergy to elastoplast or dressings, etc

in order that all staff including the chef can be informed and are aware of the problem.

Obesity

Doctors are concerned for people and particularly residents who are obese.

People who are overweight are prone to diabetes, heart attack, coronary disease and many other problems.

Unfortunately, the more obese a person becomes the more difficult it becomes to exercise (walking, swimming, etc). Due to their medical condition nursing home residents do not have as much opportunity to exercise as those in residential care homes or their own homes.

Doctors will ask for obese residents to be given a weight reducing diet until their weight falls to an acceptable level.

Unfortunately, many moderately obese residents do not accept they have a weight problem and fail to co-operate with the doctor or the staff in this matter. Some ask their friends and relatives to bring them sweets and biscuits which allows them to continue to have high calorific snacks between meals. This prevents weight loss and means they have to continue with a weight reducing diet when everybody else is having normal food.

If your relative needs a special diet of any kind, please discuss the matter with the matron and ask what delicacies, if any, you would be allowed to bring in for them.

(9)

Paying a Second Visit

If you decide to make a second visit try to take your relative with you. As it is probably going to be their new home they might like to see it before moving in. They may have questions to ask. If they can't go with you, try to discuss the options with them. This will help to make them feel they have a choice and a hand in their future.

WHY MAKE ANOTHER VISIT?

The purpose of a second visit to one of the homes on your short-list is to:

- ◆ Refresh your memory.

- ◆ Take your relative – the prospective resident – if they are willing and able.

- ◆ Clarify information you've already received.

- ◆ Ask for any more information you need.

- ◆ Have a second look at the bedrooms and communal areas.

- ◆ Discuss with the matron any changes in your relative's physical or mental health.

PREPARING FOR YOUR SECOND VISIT

1. Note any physical or mental changes in your relative, eg have they developed leg ulcers or pressure sores or been diagnosed as having an illness such as Parkinson's since you last saw the matron?

2. Note changes in their drug regime and/or treatment.

3. Phone the matron of the home and ask if there are any vacancies. Tell them of any changes in your relative's health and ask if they would still be willing to admit them.

4. If the matron agrees to admit your relative, subject to their own and the care manager's assessments, make an appointment to see the home again at a time to suit you and your relative, if they are able to go with you.

5. Prepare a new checklist and take it with you. (Don't forget to take a pen.)

See the suggested list in Figure 10. Customise it to suit the circumstances.

If you intend to visit more than one home for a second time make out another comparison chart (see Figure 11).

6. Gather together all the information about the home you are going to visit for the second time. Look through it and make a note of:

   ◆ anything you didn't ask about before

   ◆ anything you would like clarified

   ◆ new information you need.

7. Allow plenty of time for the visit.

8. Take your relative with you if possible.

9. Ask another family member or a friend to accompany you.

What to see and ask	Home 2 Ashcroft comments
Bedroom again	
Activities programme	
Church services	
Library	
Alchoholic drinks	
Smoking policy	
Pocket money	
Hairdressing – how often?	
Chiropody – how often?	
Is physiotherapy available?	
Visiting hours	
Can I bring my own furniture?	
Registered for?	
Television and licence	
Radio	
Personal insurance	
Post	
Receiving mail	
Pets	
Newspapers	
Personal laundry	
When are fees due?	
Methods of payment	
Inspection Report	
Dry cleaning	

Fig. 10. Checklist 2.

What to see and ask	Home 1	Home 2	Home 3
Bedroom again			
Activites programme			
Are there any Church services?			
Library			
Alcholic drinks			
Smoking policy			
Pocket money			
Hairdressing – how often?			
Chiropody – how often?			
Is physiotherapy available?			
Visiting hours			
Can I bring my own furniture?			
Registered for?			
Television and licence			
Radio			
Personal insurance			
Post			
Receiving mail			
Pets			
Newspapers			
Personal laundry			
When are fees due			
Methods of payment			
Inspection report			
Dry cleaning			

Fig. 11. Comparison chart for second visit.

VISITING THE SECOND TIME

◆ Introduce your relative, if they are with you, to the matron or nurse in charge.

- Ask if they can be shown a bedroom, communal rooms and bathrooms.

- Modern style baths such as a 'Parker bath' may worry your relative until they have actually tried one. Ask if your relative could see a demonstration and an explanation of how it works. They may need reassurance about any other equipment seen in the home.

- Encourage your relative to chat to staff and other residents. This will help them feel there is somebody they know in the home.

- Allow them to ask questions.

- Ask to see the menus and show them to your relative. Point out the foods you know they like.

- Ask the matron or nurse in charge to discuss the daily routine with them.

- The matron may take this opportunity to assess your relative to ensure that the home is the right place for them to be cared for on a long-term basis.

- Provided there is a vacancy most matrons will allow prospective residents to be admitted for a trial period before they decide to become a permanent resident.

- If all goes well and your relative agrees, you could ask the matron to make their assessment then, if they have not already done so, with a view to your relative's subsequent admission.

♦ If you didn't read the registration and insurance certificates, inspectors' report or the residents' charter on your last visit ask to see them.

♦ Make notes of everything you think will be important to yourself and your relative.

After the visit talk to your relative about the visit. Encourage them to see all the good things about the home. Help them to think positively about the future.

CHECKLIST

♦ Is there anything else you or your relative want to discuss?

♦ Have the assessments been carried out?

♦ Have you started to compile a list of the items they want to take with them?

10

Prior to Admission

THE MATRON'S VISIT

Before anybody can reserve a room for a prospective resident in the nursing home they feel is most suitable for them, they are usually visited by the matron or a senior member of staff. They will:

◆ Introduce themselves.

◆ Tell them more about the home.

◆ Answer any questions you or your relative may have.

◆ Discuss what you and your relative think their needs are.

◆ Make their own assessment of your relative's needs.

◆ Assess how much actual nursing care they will need.

Occasionally the matron may decide your choice of home is not appropriate for them and will refer you back to their care manager.

Reasons why a prospective resident may not be accepted

◆ It is the wrong category of home. Maybe the applicant needs a home for the mentally infirm (EMI home) or a residential care home rather than a nursing home or vice versa.

◆ The home may not be registered for the category of care your relative needs.

◆ The prospective resident may be disruptive, have behavioural problems or be excessively aggressive.

◆ There is insufficient funding.

◆ There are no vacancies.

SELF-FUNDING

Funding will depend entirely on your relative's financial status. Please look at Chapter 7.

Residents who have financial help from Social Services and are admitted to a care home of any kind will be treated exactly the same as those residents who are self-funding. In homes which have good inspection reports the quality of furniture and furnishings, decor, etc is the same in all rooms although the layout may be different due to the room's shape and size.

◆ Menus are the same for all residents except for residents who need special diets.

◆ Nursing and care may be different for individual residents, because their needs are different but the quality of care is the same for all residents.

◆ Whether a resident is self-funding or not is confidential and not generally known to anybody except the proprietor, the matron and the resident's relatives.

RESERVING A ROOM

When all the assessments and paperwork have been completed and the matron has agreed to accept your relative you will be able to reserve a room.

If your relative is self-funding they will probably be asked for a deposit which in some homes is non-returnable. The amount of deposit required is fixed by the proprietor, the managers or accountants. It may be:

◆ one week's fees
◆ one month's fees.

Ensure:

◆ you are given a receipt
◆ it is deducted from your first month's account.

PREPARING THE ROOM

The staff will:

◆ Thoroughly clean the room.

◆ Make the bed with an appropriate mattress and bedding.

◆ Check the call bell is functioning properly.

◆ Ensure a full compliment of furniture, including a commode if needed, is in place.

◆ Put towels and face cloths on the towel rails ready for use.

◆ Put a jug of fresh water within easy reach.

Personalising the room

This is an enjoyable task and the results are usually appreciated by the new resident. How you will accomplish this will largely depend on:

◆ The physical and psychological state of your relative.

◆ What your relative is allowed to take in with them.

◆ How much space is available.

◆ If the furniture can be moved around or taken out of the room.

◆ Whether your relative would like to take some of their own furniture, if this is allowed.

◆ Your relative's taste and preferences.

◆ Their interests and hobbies if any.

Some homes have the rooms redecorated in the new resident's choice of colour before admission but this is not always possible because the maintenance person may not be available to do the job. Another reason may be because many homes have a different colour scheme for various parts of the home. For instance the different floors may have a blue, green, yellow or some other colour scheme. This helps residents to know which floor they are on.

Generally speaking residents are allowed to take in small items of furniture provided it is in good condition and is free from wood worm.

Items which new residents might be allowed to take in with them:

- their favourite arm chair, providing it meets fire regulations
- a television, music centre or CD player
- books
- a limited amount of hobby and craft materials
- a clock
- pictures, paintings or photographs.

Please note: furnishings are not generally allowed because of fire regulations.

All electrical items are subject to an annual safety check by the home's own electrical contractor

INSTALLING A TELEPHONE

Most nursing and care homes have at least one pay phone for residents and staff use. Some of them are fixed on trolleys which can be brought to the resident in their room. This may be sufficient for your relative.

Ascertain whether your relative really needs a telephone in their room before you go to the expense of having one installed.

- Do they make or receive many calls?
- Would they be happy to use the trolley phone?

♦ Would they be happy to use a fixed pay phone in another part of the building?

Some homes have a system whereby the resident can make or receive calls in their own room through the home's switchboard. A charge for each call is made and added to the resident's account. Discuss this matter with the matron who will advise you.

Buying a new telephone

If your relative decides to have their own phone installed in their room, you will need to choose the one which is most suitable for them. Take into consideration:

♦ The instrument should be approved by BT and have a green label.

♦ If a phone which is not approved is purchased, BT will charge for any necessary repairs. They may also charge to correct any line faults caused by the phone.

♦ Does your relative suffer from failing sight? Look at phones with large buttons and numerals.

♦ Do they forget phone numbers easily? Look at phones with a memory.

♦ Do they have a hearing problem? BT or a hearing centre will advise on amplifiers which magnify the sound.

♦ Would your relative like to carry the phone wherever they go in the building? A cordless phone may be the answer.

♦ Personal mobile phones might not be suitable but if it seems to be the answer, check with the matron before you buy. Mobile phones may not be allowed in nursing or care homes due to the effect they might have on delicate electrical equipment.

Due to new technology it is impossible to keep up to date with all the new equipment on the market. Visit the phone shops and see for yourself what is most suitable for your relative.

DATE AND TIME OF ADMISSION

Now you and your relative have visited the homes, the choice has been made and all the assessments and the paperwork have been completed. They have decided to try it out for a fortnight. The matron has suggested a good time to admit her would be in seven days at three o'clock in the afternoon. If your relative enjoys the stay they will probably stay in the home permanently.

Arranging transport from your relative's house to the home

You will need to decide what kind of transport is required to move your relative to their new home. Do they need an ambulance? The doctor will be able to arrange it for you but there will probably be a substantial charge for this service. Look in the local phone book or ask at the surgery for names and addresses. Shop around for the best price.

If your relative can get into a car perhaps you could drive them there. If you decide on this course of action consider:

- ◆ Your car insurance – will it cover you to do this?

- ◆ Is your car suitable to transport your relative and their luggage comfortably and safely?

- ◆ Can you manage to care for them during the journey and drive as well?

- ◆ Could a friend come with you in case of an emergency?

- ◆ Could you transport them by taxi if your car breaks down?

If you decide not to drive them in your car for some reason consider:

- ◆ Can a friend with a suitable car take them, their luggage and you?

- ◆ Will your friend's insurance provide cover for all of you in the event of an accident?

- ◆ Would it be more sensible to order a taxi large enough to take both of you and the luggage?

- ◆ Some taxi firms have a vehicle suitable to transport a person sitting in a wheelchair. You might like to make enquiries.

- ◆ If absolutely necessary you can order a private ambulance but it will be costly.

- ◆ Book any transport in good time.

- ◆ Allow enough time to pack everything in a calm, unhurried manner and to make your relative comfortable for the journey.

Arranging transport from hospital to the home

If your relative is in hospital, and is to be admitted to the home from hospital, the procedure is a little different. The date and time of transfer from the hospital to the nursing home is usually arranged between the ward sister, the care manager (if appropriate) and the home. It will largely depend on the availability of hospital transport, completion of the paperwork and the most convenient time for the home to accept them. If you have a preferred time ask the ward sister if this can be taken into consideration.

RECEIVING THE CONTRACT

Either before or soon after admission your relative should receive two copies of the contract setting out terms, conditions, fees at the time of admission, details of the monthly payments and several other items of interest. It is usually a long and sometimes a complicated document.

- Read it carefully. Make sure you understand what it means.

- If in doubt ask a solicitor to unravel the jargon and interpret it for you.

- When you are completely satisfied with the contract sign both copies.

- Return one copy to the matron and keep the second copy in your file for future reference.

WHAT TO DO BEFORE ADMISSION

Make a note of all the things you need to do before your relative is admitted. It is surprising how much there is to think about and do before the day arrives.

◆ Sort out your relative's prescriptions and medications.

◆ Make a list of what medications they have and the time of day they take them.

◆ Check their clothing, replace worn out garments.

◆ Mark everything, such as clothing, glasses, television, etc.

Medications and prescriptions

If your relative is staying for a limited time ensure they have sufficient medication to last for the length of time they are going to stay in the home. It might be helpful if you can obtain a new repeat prescription from their doctor if their medications are getting low.

If your relative decides to stay permanently, the nursing or care home staff will undertake to obtain any further prescriptions and medications they will need in the future.

You may have been in the habit of dispensing their medications into containers marked out into the times and days when they are to be taken. Whilst this is an excellent way for your relative while they live alone, you must send the tablets and medicines in their original packets labelled by the dispensing chemist. The staff at their new residence will give them their medication as directed but they are not allowed to give unmarked drugs of any sort. They have to come out of the bottle or box with the name of the patient, drug and dosage clearly written on the label by the pharmacist.

Your relative's General Practitioner

Your relative may be able to remain on their current GP's list but this is not always possible. In this case your relative's name will be added to the list of the doctor who looks after the residents in the home. The doctor may not visit for a day or two after her admission and the drugs they take in with them will be used until a new prescription is issued.

Staying positive

Helping your relative to keep a positive attitude may be the hardest thing for you to cope with. Once a person has made the decision to be cared for in a nursing or care home they realise they're giving up a large part of their life. They will no longer be able to do as they like when they like. They will be leaving their house and most of their belongings, leaving the place they have made home and may have lived in for many years perhaps with their beloved spouse. Their thoughts can become negative. Instead of looking forward to good times they look back at what they had or could do years ago, when they were in their prime.

You will need to remind them they will not be lonely any more. They won't have to shop or cook for themselves, do the washing up or cleaning! Remind them they are only going to the nursing home or care home for two weeks initially and if they are unhappy they can return home. Help them to think of it as a holiday while you go away for a few days. You may find that the idea begins to regain its appeal if they think you will be away and they will be on her own for a time. Once your relative arrives in their new residence they will hopefully settle quickly and enjoy their new life. Some people adjust almost as soon as they arrive but others take a little longer to become accustomed to their new surroundings, new companions, new staff and new routine.

Sorting clothing

It's difficult to know how much or what kind of clothing another person needs. Touching their skin might give you an indication whether they are too hot or too cold, but you can't actually experience how they feel yourself.

Look at their current clothing; it will provide you with the best indication of your relative's needs and the style they like to wear.

Initially your relative will only need the amount of top clothing that they would need if they were going on holiday unless they have already made up their mind to stay in the home permanently. Even then it is better to take only the clothing you think they will want to wear during the trial period rather than everything in their wardrobe.

Choose appropriate clothing for the season, eg for summer choose a mixture, some summer clothes with some warm items because the weather is often more like winter than summer! Make sure the clothes are comfortable and still fit.

Take only as many clothes as will fit in the single wardrobe that has been provided.

As you sort through your relative's clothing discard any old and worn out items. Many elderly people neglect to renew their threadbare and torn clothes due to financial constraints. Any such essential items will need to be replaced.

Buying new clothing
When buying new clothes for your relative consider:

◆ Is it washable or dry clean only?

◆ Can it be washed in a commercial washing machine?

◆ Can it be tumble dried?

◆ Is it colour fast?

◆ Will it shrink, lose its shape or crease out of all recognition?

◆ Is thermal underwear really necessary? It doesn't always wash well in a commercial washing machine and should not be dried in a tumble drier.

◆ Consider whether your relative needs special, easy to get on clothing especially if they suffer from painful arthritis or other disability which causes pain and distress when they try to struggle into tight clothes.

Ladies		Gentlemen	
Basic underwear and nightwear			
Vests	4	Vests	4
Knickers	6 pairs	Underpants	6
Tights/stockings	6 pairs	Socks	6 pairs
Bra (if worn)	3		
Suspender belt (if worn)	3		
Corsets (if worn)	3		
Slips/half slips	4		
Nightdress/pyjamas	4	Pyjamas	4 pairs
Bed jackets	2		
Dressing gown	1	Dressing gown	1
Slippers	1 pair	Slippers	1 pair
Shoes	1 pair	Shoes	1 pair
Bed socks (if worn)	2 pairs	Bed socks (if worn)	2 pairs
Basic top clothing			
Dresses	2	Trousers	2 pairs
Skirts/trousers	2–3		
Blouses/T-shirts	3	Shirts	6
Cardigans/jumpers	3	Sweaters	2
Track suits (if preferred)	1–2	Track suits (if preferred)	1–2
For outside activities if applicable			
Coat or jacket	1	Coat or jacket	1
Hat and scarf	1	Hat and scarf	1
Gloves	1 pair	Gloves	1 pair
Outdoor shoes	1 pair	Outdoor shoes	1 pair

Fig. 12. Basic clothing required.

For a list of basic clothing see Figure 12.

Handwash and dry clean only garments

These items can get mixed up with machine washable laundry and are ruined. You may be asked to take the responsibility for this type of clothing by caring for them yourself.

If the home undertakes to send the clothes to be dry cleaned, the cost will almost certainly be added to your relative's monthly bill.

You may find the list below helpful. Each person will have their own needs so adjust the list to suit your relatives.

Buying bathroom toiletries

Favourite toiletries help to boost your relative's morale, sustain their self esteem and maintain their individuality.

The list in Figure 13 which is not exhaustive, suggests some items which you might feel are appropriate for your relative to take into the home with them.

Ladies	Gentlemen
2 face cloths (her favourite colour)	2 face cloths
2 body cloths (a different colour)	2 body cloths
Bubble bath	Bubble bath
Soap (her favourite kind)	Soap
Talcum powder	Talcum powder
Lady shaver	Razor
Nail varnish and remover	Shaving soap/cream
Antiperspirant/deodorant	Shaving brush
Cosmetics	Antiperspirant/deodorant
Body spray/perfume	Aftershave
Shampoo	Shampoo
Conditioner	Brush and comb
Brush, comb and setting aids	Toothbrush and toothpaste
Toothbrush and toothpaste	Denture cleaner if appropriate
Denture cleaner if appropriate	

Fig. 13. Suggested toiletries.

Marking personal property

Everything your relative takes with them needs to be marked, even handkerchiefs, tights or stockings, shoes and slippers. Marking clothes is more tedious and time-consuming than difficult.

Marking pen	Tends to fade with constant washing. Check often. Do clothes need re-marking?
Indian ink	Stable but can be difficult and messy to use.
Printed name tapes	Tend to fade with frequent laundering.
Tapes attached with glue	Glue does not always withstand the rigours of the washing machine. Check frequently.
Iron-on tapes	Easy to iron on but labels tend to fall off with frequent washing. Check frequently, you may need to renew them.
Woven name tapes	Some makes can be attached with special glue – see instructions. Sewing them in place takes longer but last longer. Make sure to use small stitches, if possible use a sewing machine.

♦ Get everything that needs marking together.

♦ Choose your method of marking.

♦ Check all clothing regularly. Do they need repairing or replacing?

♦ Check the name tapes frequently. Renew or re-attach when necessary.

Fig. 14. Methods of marking.

Prostheses

Prostheses are artificial parts supplied to remedy a deficiency, eg dentures. Dentures are not usually a problem to insert but a false eye may be. Everybody is different and has their own way of doing things. To eliminate any trauma or discomfort to your relative, if they use such a prosthesis ask the matron if the staff would like them or yourself (if you are able and don't mind teaching) to demonstrate the easiest and best way to insert and remove the eye prosthesis as necessary.

The same thing would apply to relatives who had any other kind of prosthesis or appliance because if they are not put on properly they will cause discomfort, soreness and pain.

Dentures	These cannot be marked satisfactorily by the general public. Your dental surgeon will advise, or go to a dental laboratory. The work will incur a charge.
Hearing aids	There are various types of these with differing amounts of space to use for marking. Either store in a marked container or you may be able to initial it with a paint pen. The supplier may be able to advise.
False eyes	Keep in a marked container or original box. These do not usually go astray.
Spectacles	Seek advice from the optician or try small self-adhesive labels.
False limbs	Try a paint pen or self-adhesive labels.
Walking aids (zimmer frame, tripod, etc)	Tie-on labels can be used but tend to disappear. Try self-adhesive labels, paint pen or a personalised walking stick badge.
Walking stick	Paint pen or personalised walking stick badge.
Wheelchairs	Large marker pen on back, self-adhesive labels or paint pen. Check name is visible frequently.
Most other items such as personal televisions, videos, helping hand radios, video or audio tapes, etc can be marked with a paint pen, marking pen or self-adhesive labels. Seek the advice of the police for more valuable items.	

Fig. 15. Ways of marking personal prostheses, equipment and property.

Some prostheses are easy to mark but dentures and eyes are not. Your relative may have containers for these items when they are not in use, which can be marked with your relative's name.

Dentures can be labelled by a skilled dental technician. There would be a charge for this but it is not a set amount. Seek advice from your dental surgeon or if this is difficult you can go direct to a dental laboratory. If your dental practice cannot supply you with the name and address of a dental laboratory you should be able to find them listed in *Yellow Pages*. You may have to go into your nearest town to find one.

Appliances and wheelchairs

All appliances and wheelchairs need to be marked. It is very easy for a walking stick or other walking aid to be accidentally left in the lounge or elsewhere. It will be returned to the person much more easily if it has the owner's name on it.

Some people have been supplied with or have purchased their own battery propelled wheelchair. You will need to enquire whether the home is suitable for one of these and whether it would be allowed. Electrical equipment, taken into a residential or nursing homes, should be checked by the home's electrical contractor to establish its safety. The matron will be able to advise whether this will apply to any electrical appliance your relative needs or wishes to take with them, eg electric pads, special beds or battery operated wheelchairs, etc.

Cigarettes and alcohol

Matron may ask for these items to be marked with the owner's name and left in the office to be given out as required. This is because some residents are not well enough to take control of them and need help when smoking or drinking alcohol. The staff will show you where the room for smokers is located if you ask them.

Please note: due to fire regulations, smoking is usually confined to a special area within the home. Smoking is not generally allowed in the bedrooms or communal areas.

Booked hospital appointments

Make two lists of any hospital appointments which have been made for your relative. The hospital will need to be notified of their change of address if they are going to be in the home on the day of the appointment. If transport has been arranged by the hospital, ask the appropriate secretary to arrange for your relative to be picked up at their new address.

The matron will need one list you have made, keep the other one for your own reference because you may like to accompany your relative to their appointment.

If you have any queries about the items your relative wants to take with them, it's advisable to ask the matron.

Pets

◆ Budgies or fish are allowed in some residential homes but the family will be responsible for their cleanliness, feeding, vaccinations and well being.

◆ Dogs and cats may be welcome to visit but they would not generally be allowed to stay.

◆ Pet tarantulas, spiders of any kind, snakes and rodents would not be welcome!

◆ Look on the contract for guidance.

You must check with the matron before bringing any animals into the home even for a visit.

Items not usually allowed

◆ Because of fire regulations residents are not usually allowed to take their own bed linen, curtains and draperies or any items of a flammable nature.

◆ Rugs and mats may cause frail elderly people to trip and fall. Therefore they are usually forbidden.

◆ Furniture which is dilapidated, dangerous or unsuitable.

Valuables

If your relative wants to take something of value into the home please:

◆ Inform the matron.

◆ Make sure the item is properly insured.

◆ Ensure jewellery can be locked away.

◆ Consider bolting Grandfather clocks or similar items to the wall.

◆ Attach paintings firmly to the wall in an inaccessible place.

A TRUE STORY

A lady was admitted to a first floor room in a nursing home. Although she was ill she was not suffering from senility. Her daughter made the room more like home, bringing photographs and pictures. One such picture was hung where the lady had full view of it and so did everybody else.

Matron was helping a care assistant to wash and dress the resident.

'Matron where has Mrs Brown's painting gone? Has her daughter taken it home?' asked the care assistant.

Matron didn't know. She phoned the daughter who denied having taken it away. The police were called in but the painting was never recovered.

The painting was a Lowry! It was very valuable and was not insured!

Reading matter

Most homes have an arrangement with the local newsagent to supply newspapers and magazines if requested. If your relative would like to take advantage of this service inform the matron or the person in charge. Ask whether you need to pay in advance or whether it will be added to your relative's account. As the arrangement may take a few days to set up you could either ask for the delivery of newspapers to commence on the day of admission, or you may prefer to supply them yourself for the first couple of days when you visit.

Library

Most homes have a library for the resident's use.

CHECKLIST

◆ Are all your relative's valuables insured?

◆ Are their clothes marked?

◆ Have you sorted out their medication?

11

Moving In

DEALING WITH EMOTIONS

New residents

It is quite common for relatives and new residents to be emotional.

Some of the things new residents may mourn the loss of include:

- their home
- their independence
- friends popping in
- carers they have made friends with
- neighbours
- the treasures they have had to dispose of
- pets they can no longer keep.

Your relative may also feel guilty because they are no longer dependent on you. Some residents feel that their carers can't exist without them leaning on them and demanding all their time.

The time inevitably comes when both of you have to start a new life.

Reassure your loved one, tell them you will visit often, do their shopping and so on.

They will appreciate your concern and realise you still care even if they won't admit it!

Relatives

Relatives who have been one of the carers or akin to a carer will almost inevitably have a feeling of guilt. They tend to tell themselves they have let their mother, father, aunt or uncle, etc down. They never think they, themselves, have become too old, too ill or too weak to care for their loved one any more. They don't believe their relative, whom they love so dearly, may now need the specialist care they cannot get at home. Every time they look at their loved one they see sadness and possibly condemnation in their eyes even if none exists. Suddenly they feel well enough to cope for a while, little thinking their own health problems will get worse for lack of proper rest, relaxation and medical attention. If you are one of these wonderful relatives or carers take heart.

If you were to become ill yourself, through continuing to care for your relative, and now you are tired and physically unable to do such strenuous work, ask yourself what would happen to your loved one if you collapsed under the constant strain of looking after them. How would you cope? How would your relative cope without you to cushion them? Try not to look back – only forward.

After the initial settling-in period your relative will probably enjoy the experience. They will never be alone. Even at night there are nurses to take them to the toilet, give them a drink, to make them a cup of tea. During the day they will have the company of other residents and will be invited to join in with any activities which have been organised.

NEW EXPERIENCES

Discuss the future with your loved one and try to discuss the clothing and other items they want to take with them including a couple of favourite pictures or photographs.

If possible take most of their luggage in beforehand so that they feel more at home when they see some of their belongings decorating their new room.

The first few times you visit them they will probably tell you of all the things that have happened to them. You will also be able to tell them what you have been doing.

It will seem strange for both of you at first. Time will go much slower than usual until you both get used to it.

Your relative will have to get used to new routines, meals at different times and eaten in a different dining area with several other people rather than somebody they love and know. Bath times will be different too.

Helping to ease the transition

When your relative's old friends fail to visit they will feel upset and neglected. Try to prevent this by:

◆ Explaining the situation to their family members, friends, fellow members of the church or clubs they attend.

◆ Giving would-be visitors their new address and phone number if they have their own telephone.

◆ Giving them the dates when they are likely to be out perhaps for a hospital appointment.

◆ Making out a visiting rota if possible.

◆ Asking the staff to encourage them to make new friends with other residents.

COPING WITH NEW ROUTINES

New places, new circumstances and new routines affect everybody differently. For some it will be getting up and bed time that will affect them most, for others it will be meals and meal times (see Chapter 9).

It will take time for your relative to get used to the people, the home, staff and everything else which is new to them. After a few days they will know some of the staff and other residents. Gradually they will begin to feel at home. Some new residents, however, take longer than others to settle in and become a valuable part of the home's community.

Dignity, privacy and independence

Loss of dignity, privacy and independence are three things which can cause fear for prospective or new residents.

Dignity (the state of being worthy of respect) is very easily destroyed but all care staff are trained to preserve the dignity and the privacy of their residents.

Independence is a little different. Most people like to do everything for themselves but sometimes what they want to do is dangerous, such as frail hands endeavouring to make a pot of tea with a heavy kettle full of boiling water.

Care staff are trained to try to eliminate dangerous ploys and to protect the residents from hurting themselves or other people. Elderly people cannot always see that something they have done all their lives has suddenly become dangerous. They feel a loss of their independence if they have to be assisted to do something they consider to be a simple job.

Visiting times

Nowadays most homes allow open visiting. That means family and friends can visit their relative at any time during the day. However, some matrons prefer visitors to visit in the afternoons and evenings so that bathing and other personal procedures can be carried out in the morning without rushing residents.

Be sure to ascertain visiting hours before you visit your relative.

Visitors

The number of visitors is not usually restricted but if the staff feel a resident is exhausted they will ask for visitors to leave in order that the resident can rest awhile.

There is one time when all visitors except for the next of kin are not allowed. This happens when the resident is seriously ill and is too sick to cope with any visitors except their nearest and dearest.

In most care homes visitors are requested to sign their name, jot down who they are visiting, the date, time of arrival and departure. This is part of the fire regulations and tells staff and fire officers who is in the building should there be a need to evacuate residents, visitors and staff for any reason.

Going out with friends or relatives

Providing your relative is well enough and the matron has given permission, you will be able to take them out. If you are going to be out for several hours, ask the nurse in charge to supply the medications your relative will need to take during the time they are out with you.

If they are incontinent you will need to ask for a supply of incontinence pads for them and it might be sensible to discreetly protect the seat of your car in case leakage occurs.

Whatever the weather, take a warm jacket or cardigan and a car blanket for them, because elderly people can feel cold even on the hottest of days.

Shopping

Your relative may ask you to take them shopping. If you agree to this make sure they don't wander off or get too tired. Some elderly people become disorientated in places like shopping malls and can get lost. To help you see them in a crowd get them to wear something bright, a scarf, belt or hat.

Make sure they have some form of identification attached to them, with their name and address and the home's phone number. If you own a mobile and have it with you, add your mobile number and make sure your mobile is ready to receive calls – just in case. If they get lost, somebody might read their details and identification and phone you with their whereabouts.

If they need a wheelchair, take their own with you.

TAKING YOUR RELATIVE ON HOLIDAY

This is quite a big undertaking but is a very worthwhile thing to do.

First you must write to the matron one month before the proposed holiday in order to:

♦ Obtain permission from the doctor.

♦ Inform the proprietors.

♦ Ensure sufficient supplies of medications have been ordered for your relative's holiday.

Give details of the proposed dates of absence, the holiday address and phone number.

If you are thinking of taking your relative abroad, ask their doctor if they are fit enough and if they need any vaccinations.

Ask for written permission from the matron to take your relative on holiday and ask for a sufficient supply of all your relative's current medications for the holiday period.

Please note:

◆ Even though your relative will not be in the home for a period of time the whole or part of the fees will still be payable in most homes.

◆ You need to take out holiday insurance for your relative as well as yourself.

If you propose travelling abroad you will need to:

◆ Ensure the air line will allow your relative to travel, with regards to health and age.

◆ Get a form E111 from the post office to cover health expenses in an emergency.

◆ Check with your travel agent if there is anything else you need to do.

Remember you will be taking full responsibility for your relative, from the time they leave the home to when they arrive back into the care of the nurse in charge again.

After the outing or holiday

Your relative may find it difficult to settle down again after a period of absence from the home, but if they are told they can go out or on holiday again, subject to their health, they will find it easier to slip back into the happy atmosphere of the home again.

(12)

Meeting New People

WHO YOUR RELATIVE WILL MEET

It can be very confusing for a new resident to move into a new home and see so many people they have never met before. Some wear uniform in different colours and styles, whilst others wear mufti.

The next few pages will give you an overview of some of the different people your relative is likely to see during their life in their new abode.

Apart from the proprietor or managers, if the home is run by a managing company, there are four main groups of people your relative may see:

◆ staff

◆ official visitors

◆ residents' visitors

◆ maintenance contractors and representatives.

The proprietor

Some proprietors visit the home at intervals, others on a regular basis which may be daily, weekly or monthly. However, many proprietors like to take an active role. If they are a Registered Nurse they may choose to become the matron of the home subject to a police check and the approval of the local Inspectors of Nursing Homes. Some proprietors prefer to be the manager, whilst others employ a firm of managers to control all aspects of the home.

Managers

If the home is run by a managerial firm, one of the team will visit periodically. They usually visit some of the residents and if there are any complaints they will discuss the matter with the complainer and endeavour to resolve the problem.

The matron

All care home employees, including the matron and nursing staff agencies, are subject to a police check. Neither the matron nor the managers are allowed to employ permanent staff who have not been vetted by the police.

Your relative may already have met either the matron, a Registered Nurse, or the matron's deputy when they were assessed prior to their admission. The matron is responsible to the proprietors and is the person who is responsible for:

◆ Dealing with enquiries regarding prospective residents.

◆ Assessing prospective residents.

◆ The admission of residents.

◆ Ensuring residents are cared for properly.

- The residents' well being.

- Engaging all or most of the staff.

- Checking the cleanliness of the home.

- Listening to and dealing with complaints.

- Proper staffing levels.

- Staff training.

- Many other things within the home.

In many homes the matron is also the manager. They may or may not wear a uniform but will usually wear a name badge.

The deputy matron

The deputy matron is a Registered Nurse and is responsible to the matron and deputises when they are not in the home. Some homes have two deputies while others have other trained and experienced staff who are able to take over when neither the matron nor the deputy are available.

The deputy matron will wear uniform and a name badge. Traditionally the uniform will be navy blue and may be a dress or trousers and top but this varies from home to home.

Some of a deputy matron's duties may include:

- Deputising for the matron when they are unavailable.

- Working with the residents.

- Being responsible for residents' well being and care.

- Supervising junior staff.

- Assisting with staff training.

- Being responsible for resident care plans and keeping them up to date.

The deputy matron's duties will inevitably overlap some of the matron's work and they will be responsible for anything the matron or the proprietor/manager asks them to do, provided it is not unlawful, is within their scope as a Registered Nurse and causes no harm to residents or staff, eg knowingly using unsafe equipment. Their duties will vary in different homes.

Registered Nurses (Sisters or Staff Nurses)

Traditionally Registered Nurses wear navy or light blue uniforms. However, many homes have their own colour scheme for their staff.

Some of the responsibilities of the Registered Nurses:

- Maintaining care of the residents.

- Teaching and supervising junior staff.

- Ensuring all the residents' care and treatment is recorded on the appropriate care plans.

- Reporting any changes in a resident's physical or mental health to the matron or the doctor.

- Dispensing prescribed drugs to the correct residents at the right time and recording this information on the residents' drug charts.

- Plus anything within reason that the matron requests.

Care assistants

Care assistants are perhaps closer to the residents than anybody else because they spend so much time caring for them.

Their main duties are:

- Assisting residents to wash or to have a bath or shower.

- Assisting residents choose their clothes for the day and to help them dress.

- Reporting to senior staff any accidents that may happen to residents.

- Reporting if residents feel or appear unwell at any time.

- Assisting residents who cannot feed themselves.

- Assisting with activities, walking, taking them to the toilet, etc.

- Preserving the residents' dignity and privacy.

- Encouraging residents to chat to each other and build up friendships.

- Helping residents undress and get ready for bed at an appropriate time for them.

- Other duties as requested by the senior staff provided it is within the boundaries of their contract and their capabilities.

The nursing staff usually work in shifts which vary slightly from home to home. They generally have two days off weekly.

Agency staff

There are occasions, perhaps due to sickness, when there is a staff shortage. If this occurs the matron has to engage temporary staff from an agency. Their uniforms may be different to the ones the permanent staff wear but they generally wear name badges.

Domestic and laundry staff

Domestic and laundry staff usually have a different coloured uniform to other staff so they are easily distinguished. They are usually given name badges to wear when they are on duty.

Domestic staff are responsible for keeping all areas of the home clean and tidy and for reporting damaged or broken furniture, etc. They would also be expected to report anything they notice about a resident which might suggest they are unwell.

In most homes laundry staff are responsible for:

- All house laundry.

- The residents' personal laundry but not their dry cleaning.

- Keeping the laundry areas and linen cupboards clean and tidy.

- Notifying the maintenance officer of machine malfunctions or breakdown.

- Informing the matron if a resident's clothing needs repairing or replacing.

- Taking the residents' clean personal laundry round to their rooms providing the items are marked with their name. (If items are unmarked they can stay in the laundry for weeks because nobody knows who they belong to.)

The maintenance officer

The maintenance officer can be either male or female so long as they are capable of carrying out the duties required by the proprietor or matron.

They usually wear some kind of protective clothing such as a boiler-suit or coloured warehouse coat.

They are responsible for:

- General maintenance of the home.

- Reporting to the matron any item needing repair.

- Arranging necessary professional help when asked by the matron.

- Carrying out minor repairs.

- Putting up shelves in residents' rooms if approved by the matron.

- Helping with moving furniture such as beds if necessary.

- Fire drills and testing fire alarms (in some homes).

- Some gardening, such as keeping paths clear of leaves, etc.

- Anything else that is requested by the matron or senior staff, providing it is within their capability and contract. This list is not exhaustive.

The gardener
Will be responsible for:

- Keeping the gardens neat and well stocked thus providing a pleasant place for residents to sit or walk.

- Planting of bulbs, seeds, plants, etc in accordance with the proprietor's or the matron's wishes.

- Mowing lawns.

- Keeping paths and areas for walking free from debris or other hazards.

- Looking after the garden tools and keeping the shed, if there is one, neat and tidy.

- Maintenance of garden furniture and garden tools/ machinery and reporting to the matron anything needing repair or replacing.

- Other jobs in the garden as designated by the management or the matron.

Residents' visitors

Residents' visitors can visit within the times stipulated by the matron or the manager. The number of residents who live in the home will determine the approximate number of visitors who come to see them.

All visitors are required to sign in the visitor's book both when they arrive and when they leave the home. This is to comply with fire regulations.

General Practitioners and Consultants

Doctors visit to make routine checks on their patient's progress or deterioration or if they are called in by the nursing staff.

Consultants will make domiciliary visits if requested by the doctor.

Hairdresser/barber

Some homes have their own hairdressing salon and in larger establishments a hairdresser may attend on a part-time basis. In smaller homes a visiting hairdresser will either use the resident's room or some other designated place to attend to the hairdressing needs of residents.

Nowadays, the ladies' hairdressers will also attend to men's hair. This is very useful because it is not always easy to engage a barber to trim the men's hair for them.

The matron will arrange for a hairdresser to visit regularly, weekly or fortnightly.

Chiropodist

The matron usually arranges for a chiropodist to treat all residents' feet that need attention. They hold their 'clinic' either in a designated place or they will visit residents in their own rooms.

Opticians

If your relative has a problem with their sight ask the matron if you can take them to an optician (if that is practical) or if they can arrange for an optician to make a domiciliary visit to carry out an examination of their eyes.

Vicars, priests and other church leaders

Church services are held in many homes now. If your relative belonged to an Anglican or Roman Catholic church prior to admission they will almost certainly be able to participate in a suitable 'church service' held by an appropriate church leader.

Residents who used to attend a Baptist, Methodist, United Reform, Pentecostal or a church of a different denomination, are usually asked if they would like to participate in an inter-denominational church service. Such services are often held within the home by one of the pastors.

There are organisations, eg PARCHE, which send dedicated Christian volunteers into care homes to organise short inter-denominational services for residents and their visitors. After the service the volunteers usually wander round and talk to the residents before they leave.

OFFICIAL VISITORS

The main groups of official visitors who visit the home are:

◆ inspectors
◆ district pharmacist
◆ fire officer
◆ police officers
◆ ambulance crews and paramedics
◆ maintenance contractors.

Inspectors

Care home inspections are carried out four times a year. Extra inspections may be carried out if the inspectors are dissatisfied with any aspect of the running of the home, eg management or the residents' well being.

The purpose of their inspection is to:

◆ Ensure the well being of the residents.

◆ Assess whether residents are contented, happy and well looked after.

◆ Ensure the mix of staff and staffing levels are adequate.

◆ Ensure the home is being run in a proper manner.

◆ Check all records are updated regularly.

◆ Check residents' personal care plans are accurate and revised whenever there is a change in the resident's physical or mental condition, care or treatment.

◆ Check the cleanliness of the kitchen(s).

- See menus are well balanced, nutritious and appetising.

- Check all parts of the home are being kept clean.

- Check all table linen, bed linen and residents' clothing is laundered as necessary.

- See anything else they wish to.

Two of the inspections are unannounced but the inspectors make appointments with the matron for the other two. This is because they need to see all the records, care plans, etc on these visits.

It is an ideal time for residents to chat to the inspectors, particularly if they have a complaint, suggestions or want to give praise!

The district pharmacist
The district pharmacist may not be seen by the residents as they will spend their visit checking all the drugs (medications) in the home.

Some of the things they will check are:

- The expiry date on all drugs and medications.

- Tablets, creams, ointments, medicines, etc are stored in a proper manner.

- New stocks are checked and recorded both when they arrive and when they are dispensed to the appropriate resident.

- Residents' drug charts are kept up to date.

Fire officers
Fire officers visit from time to time and your relative may see them checking fire extinguishers, fire hoses, smoke and fire alarms which are placed in strategic places around the home.

They will also check fire exits to make sure they are uncluttered as this could prevent a safe exit in the event of a fire.

The fire records will be inspected for frequency of staff fire training and testing of fire equipment.

Police officers
Police officers will attend if they are called by the management, the matron or senior staff in the event of burglary, theft or other crime being committed on the premises.

Ambulance crews and paramedics
Ambulances with paramedics will be called into the home in the case of sudden illness or an accident to a resident or member of staff.

Hospital transport vehicles will attend to take a resident to the hospital for a hospital appointment if required.

Maintenance contractors
Maintenance contractors carry out inspections and repairs to equipment or to the building when called in by the management.

Lifts have to be inspected at regular intervals by the manufacturer's own maintenance team or another firm as arranged by them.

In the event of a breakdown they will be called out by the nurse in charge to carry out urgent repairs.

MOVING

Changing rooms
If for any reason your relative is moved into another room, all their belongings, including pictures and ornaments, will be taken into the new room by staff. You may find the handyman, whom they might not have seen before, is helping. Tell them not to be alarmed, the staff will not change, only the room.

Changing homes
Unfortunately, sometimes residents have to go into hospital for a few days. All the staff will be different, with different uniforms, different names and so on. However, once they are well again they will most likely be transferred back to the care home they are used to.

If your relative has been transferred to hospital for a serious illness or surgery, they will need nursing care and may not be able to return to the residential care home where they may have been for a long time. In a case like this your relative would be placed in a nursing home. Staff, uniforms, routines and many other things would be different.

It is not unusual, after traumatic changes like this, for elderly people to become confused, tearful and possibly depressed for a time. They will gradually feel better as they make new friends. However, this may take time because an elderly person often takes longer to recover from a serious illness or surgery. Your relative may become demanding, sorry for themselves (with good reason) and will need much understanding, comforting and tender loving care.

Overcoming Difficulties

STRESS

Experts tell us that moving house is one of the most stressful events in a person's life. Unfortunately, moving a relative from their home into a care home on a permanent basis is not only very stressful for them but it also affects you and the rest of the close family.

Understanding your relative's stress

Try to remember their stress may cause fluctuating mood changes. One day they may be feeling happy, they like the idea of going into a nursing home; all their thoughts are positive. The next day they may be down in the dumps. They hate the thought of going into a nursing home, they would rather die!

To help to relieve your relative's stress before admission you can:

◆ Talk to your relative in a positive way.

◆ Emphasise the disadvantages of them staying in their own home.

◆ Take them, if possible, to see the home.

◆ Point out all the advantages of living in such a place.

- When the matron comes to assess their prospective resident, encourage your relative to ask questions.

- Discuss every step and every aspect with them.

- Keep them informed.

- Encourage them to help in the preparation for their move to their new home.

- If possible arrange a trial period before making a permanent commitment.

- Tell your relative that some of their treasures are already in their new home ready for them.

Beating your own stress

If you are the person who made all the arrangements for your relative to be admitted into the home, you will most likely suffer from more stress than the rest of the family. You might worry that things will go wrong or your relative will be unhappy; they will not like the staff or the staff won't like them. All the things that could go wrong, and probably won't, churn around in your mind chasing positive thoughts away. This is worse if your relative grumbles about their changed circumstances, blaming you for putting them in this 'dreadful situation'! At this stage they will forget they couldn't take themselves to the bathroom or that they need help with all the activities of daily living. They won't admit that in the times when they are alone, particularly in the night hours, they sometimes feel lonely and afraid.

It is useless to tell you not to take any notice or to forget the hurt because it won't work. However, take time off to:

- Relax, you might like to join a relaxation class.

- Try a keep fit or dancing class. Exercise boosts the morale.

- Read, watch television, cat-nap or anything else you fancy for an hour.

- Try prayer: many people find comfort and peace in it.

- Chat with a minister of religion. It may help put things into perspective.

- Talk over the problems with somebody else. Perhaps a friend has gone through the same experience and can offer helpful advice.

- Discuss everything, good and bad, with other family members – let them shoulder some of the responsibility.

- Try to draw up a visiting rota between family and friends to give you more time and relieve some of your stress and anxiety.

GRIEVING

Your relative is probably grieving. It's hard for an elderly person to give up their home and most or all of their possessions, go into a strange place and live a totally different life style.

It comes as a shock to elderly people to find they need help with personal and intimate care, they find it very embarrassing to have to rely on young nurses to take them to the toilet or help them sit on a commode, especially if they are of the opposite sex, and they grieve for what they have lost.

Grieving can make them:

♦ Frustrated because nobody believes they could still care for themselves in their own home.

♦ Sad and weepy.

♦ Feel worthless and isolated.

♦ Depressed.

♦ Fear the loss of freedom and independence.

♦ Suicidal.

Grieving can lead to:

♦ discontentment
♦ loss of interest
♦ loss of appetite
♦ weight loss
♦ tearfulness
♦ sickness
♦ aggression
♦ depression.

Wanting to go home

Anxiety and stress can start before your relative is ever admitted to a care home. If they have been ill and have been treated in hospital they will be longing to go home. Then they are told they are going to be transferred into a nursing home. They have received a shock. They want to go home and can't understand why other people think they need to be looked after. They don't realise they are weaker now and can't do the things they were once capable of.

Recuperating in a nursing home may show them they need more help now they are older or since they have been ill or because of their frailty – which they hadn't noticed before.

They may begin to wonder how they could manage to cope without being able to call somebody to help them get to the bathroom, dress and to get their meals. Recognising their current needs and lack of ability may well be another reason for them to grieve for the health and strength they once had.

If they can be persuaded to adopt a more positive attitude they will become more contented, helpful and co-operative. Changing a person's attitude will take time and can be wearing on their visitors but when they have settled and you see a smile on their face again, you will realise it has all been worth while. Their outlook on life and health will improve and they will become more contented and possibly will want to join in some of the organised activities. They will have hope and begin to enjoy life in their new home.

MOVING IN – THE FIRST FEW HOURS

If you cannot take your relative to the home where they are being admitted, it would help them if you could be there when they arrive.

On arrival your relative will be greeted and made welcome. The nurse will probably offer them and their relative refreshments. They will be shown to their room and made comfortable.

Soon afterwards a nurse will introduce themselves and chat whilst filling in an admission sheet. This is a good time to ask any questions and the nurse will take your relative to the toilet if necessary.

Later, your relative's temperature, pulse, respiration and blood pressure might be taken. The nurse may ask for a urine sample for testing. When they are getting ready for bed the nurse will note if they have any skin damage such as:

- redness of the skin
- bed sores
- bruising from falling
- cuts and abrasions.

They will be weighed soon after admission.

These simple tests and observations are carried out to ensure whether or not new residents are suffering from any obvious condition which needs treatment. The results occasionally lead the nurse to suspect there could be a problem. This would be monitored and reported to the doctor. However, most findings are normal and are used as a base line.

New residents will, at some point, have their photo taken for identification purposes. This is particularly helpful for new staff. The chef, if available, may come and discuss the menu with them. Staff will come as soon as possible to unpack their belongings and put them away. Afterwards, depending on the time, they may be taken into the lounge or dining room and introduced to other residents. Bedtime is variable depending on each resident's preference.

Some ways to help relieve stress after admission

◆ Encourage their friends to visit and reassure them they will continue visiting.

◆ Visit as often as you can, even though it might be discouraging at first.

◆ Take in small gifts, eg a tablet of their favourite soap.

◆ Encourage them to make friends with other residents.

◆ If possible take them out for an hour or two, perhaps in a wheelchair.

◆ Tell them how much better they look.

◆ Take them some flowers.

◆ Spend time chatting to them over a cup of tea.

CHANGING ROUTINES

Your relative may be or have been married, widowed or they may have chosen to remain single. They will most likely have been living in their own home either with their partner or by themselves for a long time. Over the years they will have developed their own pattern of living, for instance they may have been getting up at 6 every morning and going to bed at 9 each night. Meals would have been be prepared and eaten at a time which fitted into their lifestyle.

Although all care homes have their own routine they are not inflexible. Generally speaking, residents can have an early morning cup of tea, rise at the time they prefer and go to bed when they choose.

Meal times are usually at set times but do not often cause a problem. If the evening meal clashes with their favourite television programme ask the staff if it can be served in their room.

The luxury of a bath

Active and able people have a bath or shower whenever it suits them, sometimes two or even three times a day. They take a bath without any further thought.

Elderly and disabled people are not as able to have a bath or shower as often as they used to due to difficulties caused by their disabilities. Some seldom get into the bath but content themselves with a good wash when they need one.

In a care home a bath can become a luxury. Some homes endeavour to give every resident a bath or shower every day if it is appropriate for them. However, this is not always possible and residents are allocated bath days. This allows the resident to have more time for their bath and feel relaxed rather than rushed. If the allocated days are not suitable for your relative, ask if they can be changed to a more preferable day or time.

Specialist baths are fitted in most homes. Some of them look different to what your relative will have been used to and they may even be nervous of using them.

They have no need to be afraid, there will always be a nurse with them to help them get in and out of the bath, to wash, dry and dress themselves.

Needing spiritual fellowship

If your relative is a practising member of a church they will miss the fellowship and friendship of other church members. Contact their vicar, pastor or church leader. They may be able to arrange regular visits from the church pastoral team. They may also be able to arrange occasional church meetings within the home subject to the matron's agreement.

Many church leaders already conduct meetings in homes for the elderly. The date and time of such services are usually pinned to the notice board. If you can't find the information you need, the matron will be able to give you the date of the next meeting, if one has already been arranged.

MAKING COMPLAINTS

Occasionally your relative has something they cannot cope with any longer. For instance, it may be loud music from somebody's television. Ask one of the nurses if they could persuade the resident to turn down the volume to a more acceptable level. If there is no change you or your relative might like to make an official complaint. Start by speaking to the nurse in charge or the matron. If nothing is done speak to your relative's care manager if they have one, or to the manager or proprietor.

If nothing is done about the complaint write a letter to the manager or proprietor telling them no action has been taken. Suggest that they might like to visit the room and hear the noise for themselves.

Should your letter be ignored send a reminder. If you do not get a satisfactory solution to the problem write to the inspector of the home who will investigate the problem (see Figure 16).

1. Make your complaint to the **nurse in charge**.
2. If no change complain to the **matron**.
3. Still no change: speak to the **Care Manager**.
4. No response: speak to the **manager or proprietor**.
5. Complaint ignored: put it in writing to the **manager or proprietor**.
6. Complaint still ignored: send a reminder to the **proprietor**.
7. Still no response: write to the **Nursing Home Inspector**.
8. The **Inspector** will:
   ◆ Investigate the complaint.
   ◆ Discuss it with the matron.
   ◆ Discuss it with the proprietor.
   ◆ Problem solved.

Fig. 16. Making a complaint.

Things You Need to Know

USEFUL INFORMATION

Television licence

If your relative takes their own television into the home, they will be required to buy their own television licence unless they are over the age of 75 years. However, their current licence is transferable when they move to another home. Please verify this with the matron or the manager.

Car insurance

Make sure your car insurance covers any passengers from the home you choose to take on an outing.

Special occasions

Don't forget to inform the matron in writing if you intend to take your relative out or prepare something special for their birthday or Christmas. Ensure you have their permission before you finalise your plans.

Reading matter

If there are no library services within the home, go to your local library and borrow books or tapes for your relative. The borrower (yourself) will be responsible for the borrowed book or tapes and for them being returned on time in good condition.

Getting some fresh air

Take your relative out for a ride, or a walk, or in a wheelchair if they are not mobile. Make sure you notify the staff and record it in the visitors' book.

Bedsores, leg ulcers and dressings

Your relative's doctor will prescribe treatment for leg ulcers, bed sores and all other skin problems. Treatment will be carried out by the registered nurses in nursing homes. If your relative has had to change their doctor since being admitted to a home the treatment prescribed by the new doctor may be different to what they are used to.

If your relative has been admitted to a residential care home, the treatment will be carried out by the community nurses.

Accidents and sickness

If your relative has an accident or becomes sick, the doctor will be informed. They will visit if it is deemed necessary.

If a fall has caused concussion or they have sustained a fracture they will be sent by ambulance to the nearest accident and emergency department for diagnosis. If necessary they will be admitted for observation and treatment.

The nurse in charge will do their best to inform you of the situation and give you the opportunity to accompany your relative in the ambulance.

Blood tests

If your relative's doctor wants them to have a blood test they will either take the blood or ask a registered nurse to do so. If your relative resides in a residential care home the community nurse will be asked to take their blood and send it to the lab.

Bedtime

Is your relative warm enough in bed at night? Ask for an extra blanket for them if required. Extra pillows will be provided if they need them. It is possible they may need warmer night wear and bed socks.

Check clothing

Check your relative's clothing at the beginning of each season to ensure they have a suitable range of clothing to match the weather.

A shawl is useful for chilly evenings. Gloves, scarves, a hat and warm shoes will be needed for outings during winter weather.

Short of cash?

Look round the local charity shops for good quality clothing, jigsaw puzzles and books at reasonable prices. Be discerning, examine everything before you actually buy.

Calendar

Buy a large calendar to hang on the wall. Note special events, birthdays, etc on the appropriate date as a reminder. Help them buy and write cards and undertake to post them.

Post

Ask the matron what the postal arrangements are. Most homes have a letter box for the residents' outgoing mail, it will then be taken by a member of staff and posted.

Residents' mail is delivered to the home, provided it's addressed properly.

It will then be delivered to the residents by a member of staff.

Phone numbers

Give your relative an address book with the address and phone numbers of all her friends.

Magnetic boards

A magnetic board is a good idea to hold photos, messages, memos, etc.

Advice

Ask your relative's advice sometimes. It will make them feel useful and wanted.

Carrying bits and pieces

Make them a bag that can be attached to their zimmer walking aid. If they don't use a zimmer make them an apron with a large pocket, big enough to hold the things they always want to carry with them. Handbags get left behind and are easily lost, aprons will stay attached to them.

Lockable safe, cupboard or drawer
Residents should be provided with a facility for keeping private papers, small amounts of money, etc either in a lockable top drawer or cupboard. If none are provided, ask the matron if they can get a lockable facility fitted.

If your relative has a lot of cash with them, it must be handed over to the matron or nurse in charge to be kept in the home's safe. Make sure you get a receipt for the cash.

Visitor's rota
- Arrange visiting times with your relatives and friends.

- Make out a visitors' rota.

- Enter the days and times they are expected on your relative's calendar.

- Remember visitors may be restricted if your relative becomes too ill or frail to cope with more than one or two at their bedside.

Newspapers
Spend some time reading the newspaper to them. It can be quite tiring for an elderly person to hold up a newspaper for any length of time, particularly the broad sheets.

Local papers may be of more interest to them because they will probably know the area and possibly some of the people, especially if they have lived there for a long time.

SPIRIT LIFTERS

♦ Bring in a nail care kit and give your relative a manicure.

♦ Make up a scrap book of comic strips found in some of the daily papers.

♦ Make another scrap book with puzzles, word games, and crosswords. Cut them out from the daily papers or magazines. It's even better if you can get the answers which usually appear in the following day's paper.

♦ Painting is a very therapeutic pastime. Your relative might like to have a painting by numbers set.

♦ Bring their pet to visit if they have one, but obtain the matron's permission first.

♦ Some ladies are delighted with a perfume spray, it makes them feel special.

♦ Many people like to do jigsaw puzzles. Get a reasonably small one that's not too complicated to start with.

♦ If they enjoy this pastime you might like to get them a jigsaw roll which rolls up with the puzzle inside. The jigsaw remains as it was left and pieces stay intact. Don't buy one until you're sure they will use it.

♦ In hot weather a fan would be appreciated. A cooling cologne stick is also welcome.

♦ Lavender bags will keep clothing and drawers smelling nice.

♦ Provided your relative is not on any special diet or is diabetic, they might like to have a dish of wrapped sweets in their room. Some residents enjoy offering staff a sweet when they come in to attend to them.

◆ Your relative may appreciate some flowers providing they are not allergic to them. Sweet smelling freesias perfume the room. Most homes seem to be short of vases, bring an inexpensive vase for them. Don't forget to mark the vase with their name.

◆ Christian folk love to have passages from the Bible read to them. They often have favourite readings, such as the Psalms. They might appreciate it if you read a few verses to them. Alternatively you could borrow from the library or buy them an audio tape or CD of sacred music or passages from the Bible from a Scripture or Bible shop. Make sure they have the right equipment to play it. A Walkman type of machine could be useful.

DETERIORATION OF HEALTH AND DYING

You will be called if your relative's health deteriorates and given the option of visiting. The doctor will be notified of the deterioration and may visit, depending on when they last examined them. A nurse is usually detailed to sit with them.

When their pulse and respiration has ceased and they appear to have passed away, the doctor will be notified and will come to certify death as soon as possible. Sometimes the doctor will write the death certificate at the time or may leave it at the surgery for you to pick up.

All the details of their wishes should have been recorded in their notes at the time of admission.

Your relative's contract should tell you the number of days you have to clear the room of all their personal belongings without extra charges being incurred.

If your relative has been allowed to have a pet, it will have to be removed after their death unless the matron decides it could stay at the home for the benefit of the other residents.

What happens when my relative dies?
The procedure will be different if your relative is not a Protestant.

If they are of the Jewish faith, the Rabbi must be notified when death is imminent. They will make all the arrangements for attending to them and their removal when the time comes. In a case like this the staff are not allowed to touch them after they have passed away, unless specific instructions have been given. A similar situation arises in some other religions. It is essential for you to have given the matron details of your relative's requirements at the time of their admission.

After the doctor has certified death, your relative will be taken by the undertaker of your choice to a chapel of rest until the death certificate and further instructions from the next of kin have been received.

The room will have to be cleared and all accounts settled within a given time (see the contract).

Some matrons like to send somebody to the funeral to represent the home and would be grateful if you notify them of the date, time and place where this will be held.

MRS WINTERS' STORY

Mrs Winters was sitting in the office having a cup of tea when I arrived.

'I wondered if you had any rooms vacant Matron,' she asked.

'Yes, there is an empty room on the top floor. Can you tell me why you're interested in it?'

'My aunt aged 70 is still in hospital, she's just had a fall and broken her hip. The surgeon has put a new hip joint in and she is going to be discharged soon.'

I asked her some questions about her aunt and then spoke about the home. When she had drunk her tea we went upstairs to look at the vacant room.

We were in the new wing of the building, it hadn't been in use very long.

The room looked lovely with the sun shining in through the windows. Mrs Winters thought it would be just right for her aunt.

We went down to the office again and I filled in an application form for her.

'Is there anything you would like to ask me or is there anything you would like to see?'

'How much will it cost for a week?'

Mrs Winter was nervous because she had to persuade her aunt to recuperate in a nursing home for a few weeks. She knew her aunt could afford to pay the fees but was unsure whether she would spend a large sum of money on herself.

'Have you a cheaper room?' she asked hesitantly.

'I'm sorry we haven't anything less than £500 a week I'm afraid, we charge the same amount for all our rooms.'

'I don't know what my aunt will say.'

'Why don't you look around at other nursing homes, maybe somebody will have a less expensive room than the one you've just seen.'

'I don't really want to because I like that room upstairs. Perhaps I ought to see what my aunt thinks.'

Mrs Winters went back to the hospital and I didn't see her for several days. She looked tired.

'How can I help you today Mrs Winters?'

'I saw my aunt and she grumbled at me and sent me to every other home to see if there was anywhere cheaper, but there wasn't.' 'So I've come back here again. My aunt wants to see you as soon as possible. She really would like that room upstairs because I've told her so much about this place – and that room.'

I did visit Mrs Winters' aunt the following day. She was enthusiastic and wanted to be discharged as soon as possible. She thrust a cheque into my hand for the deposit after I said she could be admitted to our home.

Mrs Winters' aunt was admitted as soon as she was fit enough to leave the hospital. She was a very amenable lady who, like most people, expected value for her money. She soon settled down and stayed with us for several weeks. Before she left she told us she would return when she could no longer live alone in her own home.

Lessons to be learned

When interviewing a person who is a prospective resident or who wants a room for a relative or friend, it is helpful to give accurate answers to all the questions they ask. However, when I was a matron many people who visited and wanted to find out more seemed to be a little overcome and often forgot all the questions they really wanted to ask. If only they had made a list of all their queries it would have been much easier for them.

Useful Addresses

Age Concern London, 54 Knatchbull Road, London SE5 9QY. Tel: 020 7737 3456

Aid for the Aged in Distress, 54 London Road (CCUK), Morden, Surrey SM4 5BE. Tel: 013 4271 8524

Alzheimer's Society, Gordon House, 10 Greencoat Place, London SW1P 1PH. Tel: 020 7306 0606

Arthritis Association, I Upperton Gardens, Eastbourne, East Sussex. Tel: 01323 416550

Arthritis Care, 18 Stephenson Way, London NW1 2HD. Tel: 020 7386500

British Heart Foundation, 14 Fitzharding Street, London W1H 4DH. Tel: 020 7935 0185

Chaseley Trust, South Cliff, Eastbourne, East Sussex BN20 7JH. Tel: 01323 744200

Diabetes UK, 10 Parkway, London NW1 7AA. Tel: 020 7424 1000

Greater London Fund for the Blind, Dept. CC, 12 Whitehorse Mews, London SE1 7QD. Tel: 020 7620 2066

Help the Aged, St James's Walk, Clerkenwell Green, London EC1R 0253. Tel: 020 7253 0253 Free Information Line: 0808 800 6565

MIND (National Association for Mental Health), Granta House, 15–19 Broadway, London E15 4BQ

Mind Information Line: 08457 660 163 (9.15am–5.15pm)

Parkinson's Disease Society (Head Office), 215 Vauxhall Bridge Road, London SW1. Tel: 020 7931 8080 National Help Line: 0808 800 0303

Stroke Association, Stroke House, White Cross Street, London EC1Y 8JJ. Tel: 020 7516 0300

Useful Web Sites

ONLINE DATABASES

www.bettercaring.co.uk
Offers searchable database of all registered Care Homes in UK (over 20,000 listed) with more than 4 beds. Uses BEDVACS facility – constantly updated online database of bed availability.

www.bupa-carehomes.co.uk
BUPA Care Homes is the largest and most acknowledged Nursing Home provider in the UK. BUPA Care Homes manages over 245 homes around the county, caring for over 15,000 residents.

www.carehomes.uk
Over 17,000 Care Homes (and care homes w/nursing) in the UK.

www.carehomesuk.net
Largest online database of Care Homes; nursing and residential homes, hospices and respite homes. Links to websites of individual Care Homes.

www.nursinghomes.co.uk
NHS Registry – Registered nursing, rest, retirement, warden-assisted, respite, convalescent, elderly and special care homes, listed in full detail by UK region.

www.ucarewecare.com
UK Nursing Homes Directory (nursing homes, financial advisers and care agencies).

GENERAL INFORMATION
www.british services.co.uk/nursinghomes.htm
Govt bodies/institutions/associations and resources – lists further sites.

www.carestandards.gov.uk
National Care Standards Commission website.

www.care-solution.co.uk
Nursing Homes and other care; comprehensive advice and solutions.

www.doh.gov.uk/ncsc/carehomesolderpeople.pdf
Dept of Health – Care Standards Act 2000.

www.housingcare.org
A site for older people and all who provide housing, care or support to them. Helping to make decisions about where to live and any support/care required.

www.saga.co.uk/health_news/pages/resource_centre.asp? Iss = accommodation
Saga Health Resource Centre; links to numerous websites concerned with nursing care and accommodation.

www.thepensionservice.gov.uk/atoz/atozdetailed/rescare. asp
The Pension Service – Part of Dept for Work and Pensions (going into a care home, how to pay costs, more info, other help).

FINANCIAL ADVICE

www.bettercaring.co.uk

Links to two specialist Financial Advisers (NHFA and Care Aware); free advice on care funding, regardless of financial circumstances. Confirm eligibility for State assistance to contribute to cost of care.

www.carefeesinvestment.co.uk

Care Home fees planning; Residential Care costs planning.

www.capitalcare.co.uk

Care Homes fees payment options.

www.nhfa.co.uk

(Nursing Home Fees Agency). Free advice and information about getting and paying for care.

www.sofa.org

Online search facility; find an IFA to help with advice about paying for and co-ordinating long-term care.

MISCELLANEOUS

www.careshow.co.uk

The annual care show at Bournemouth International Centre is dedicated to the nursing and care home business but also to people with mobility problems and their carers. The exhibition is usually held in March or April. Check the website for dates.

Index